Sweat

Sweat

A History of Exercise

Bill Hayes

BLOOMSBURY PUBLISHING

NEW YORK · LONDON · OXFORD · NEW DELHI · SYDNEY

BLOOMSBURY PUBLISHING
Bloomsbury Publishing Inc.
1385 Broadway, New York, NY 10018, USA

BLOOMSBURY, BLOOMSBURY PUBLISHING, and the Diana logo are
trademarks of Bloomsbury Publishing Plc

First published in the United States 2022

LIBRARY OF CONGRESS CATALOGING-IN-PUBLICATION DATA IS AVAILABLE

ISBN: HB: 978-1-62040-228-3; EBOOK: 978-1-62040-229-0

2 4 6 8 10 9 7 5 3 1

Typeset by Westchester Publishing Services
Printed and bound in the U.S.A.

To find out more about our authors and books visit www.bloomsbury.com and
sign up for our newsletters.

Bloomsbury books may be purchased for business or promotional use. For information
on bulk purchases please contact Macmillan Corporate and Premium Sales
Department at specialmarkets@macmillan.com.

CONTENTS

The immortal gods have made it so:
To achieve excellence, we first must sweat.

—HESIOD, *WORKS AND DAYS*, CA. 700 B.C.

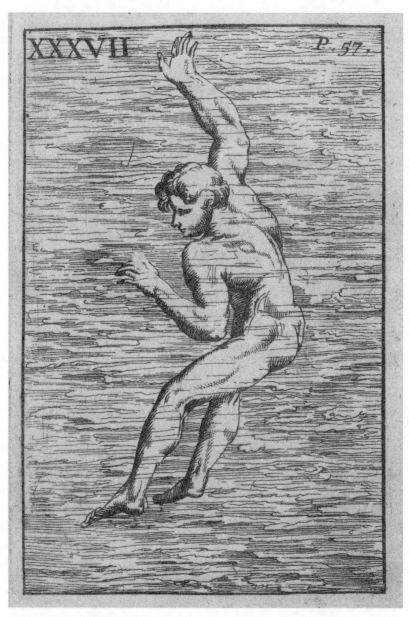

From *L'Art de nager (The Art of Swimming)* by Melchisédech Thévenot, 1696;
one of the earliest instructional manuals on swimming

Plunge

My body has no idea what is about to happen. No idea. I take off my shirt and shorts, my shoes. I sit. I am ready, but still I wait. I am preparing myself, or think I am, but cannot. I look into the water, as if for a sign. There is none. And then something urges me forward—resignation, or impatience, or maybe it's merely that the dock flies are biting me—and I push off. There is violence in this: the body breaking the glassy surface, crashing through it, the blasting noise in one's ears—and the feeling on one's skin, *of* one's skin and nerves, down to the bones. It is a sensation not unlike pain.

I suppose it is pain. I think of icicles breaking. There is sharpness. I have my goggles on and see what I feel: chaos, a watery chaos, a chaos of sensations. Murky greens and browns and blacks and also splashes of white, like slashes of paint, through the transparency, through the vitreous of the eye of the lake. I see my arms akimbo before me, and bubbles—air bubbles. I feel like a scuba diver with no gear, and there is a flash of panic; the water is cold, fifty degrees I'm told, and I am almost confused by it, the not-rightness of it. But in that same instant, I am moving forward, pushing through the water, onward.

I kick hard, instinctively feeling that by kicking I will get away from the cold. There is nothing else to do. Now I see my arms stretched out before me, my hands in a V, and I am bulleting through the water, conscious that I am moving—flying—and that the air in my lungs is running out.

I see the green transparency lightening, the surface nearing. I reach my right hand forward as far as I can and my left arm back, as if pulling the string on a bow, in position to launch into freestyle as soon as I emerge.

Surfacing is the opposite of plunging, but it feels the same, the huge chaos of sensations—sensations of temperature, water, force, light. Yes, now there is light as I break through and see the shore, the boathouse, trees, and I grab for air (that's how it feels, *gasp* is not the right word, it has a physical, muscular feeling to it), grab a lungful, and thrust, pull, kick, rotate: swim. I go as far as four or five breaths will take me, as far as I can go without thinking of anything else, then turn around. Climbing onto the dock, my skin and muscles are taut, oxygenated.

Later, a friend asks me why I would do this—it's October, for God's sake; the lake is freezing.

"Because I can," I say.

SOMEONE ONCE TOLD me that the American composer Virgil Thomson, on turning ninety, said that he was happy at last because now he no longer had to take any exercise. (He lived two more presumably exercise-free years.) This would not be my attitude. One of my big fears about getting old is that I won't be able to get any exercise at all—that I'll be stuck in front of a TV, bedridden, not able to lift, run, take a walk. Please, shoot me first. No, wait. Throw me into a lake. I want to go out swimming when the time comes.

It's in my DNA in some way, this desire for the physical. From as young as twelve or thirteen, I had a keen interest in the human body, which led me later in life to write books about the science of sleep, the history of human blood, and the story behind the classic nineteenth-century text *Gray's Anatomy*. For this, I spent a year studying anatomy alongside first-year med students, doing full cadaver dissection and trying to get a feel for what the original Henry Gray had done. After finishing that book, I had time on my hands and spent hours working out at a gym, running, going to yoga and spin classes. Exercise and I had a long history by this point, yet the notion that exercise itself might have a history—that there could be such a thing—never occurred to me until one afternoon at the gym about twelve years ago.

I climbed atop a StairMaster, long my cardio machine of choice, both because it kicks your butt and gives you a certain psychological lift—you are a good four feet taller than those on the floor and feel like you can conquer anything. I punched in my usual program—Fat Burner, level 15, at twenty-five minutes. I arranged my towel and bottle of water, and thumbed in my iPod earphones. My finger found the machine's START button, that small green circle, so powerfully endowed; each time you press it is a chance to wipe the slate clean and absolve yourself of somatic sins. Yet for some reason, I hesitated a moment on this particular day. I took in the scene before me—men and women of all ages and diverse origins, lifting weights, back-bending over giant rubber balls, fitting themselves into torturous-looking apparatuses, pulling themselves up on chin-up bars—and a thought popped into my head: *How did we all end up here? If I were to trace a line back in time to the beginnings of exercise, where would I land?*

I stood there and thought for a long while before pressing CLEAR, then took up my towel and water and climbed back down. What I did next was pure reflex: I went to the library.

LIBRARIES, LIKE GYMS, have always been a refuge for me, just as gyms, like libraries, have always been places of learning. I started poking around. I found lots of listings in the card catalog for health and exercise manuals—most from the present day, but also a surprising number from the nineteenth century and earlier. The titles were tantalizing: *Exercising in Bed*; *Man, the Masterpiece*; and a mouthful from 1796, *An Easy Way to Prolong Life, By a Little Attention to Our Manner of Living, Containing Many Salutary Observations, on Exercise, Rest, Sleep, Evacuations, etc.*, whose author was listed only as "Medical Gentleman."

Unfortunately, all these old volumes were long lost or missing, and I didn't find a book that succinctly answered my question about the origins of exercise. That was that; I didn't pursue it further, as other concerns soon took over. I decided to move to New York, something I had wanted to do since I was a kid. I felt that it was now or never, so at age forty-eight, in the spring of 2009, I started my life over. I got a full-time job. I fell in love with my late partner, the neurologist and author Oliver Sacks. I got to know the city. I lived on the West Side of Manhattan for a year, then on the East, then moved back to the West. I had a full-time job and didn't have much time for writing, although I always had time for working out. I belonged to seven different gyms in a three-year period until I found one with which I shared the right chemistry. It is a physical relationship, after all.

Every now and then in my reading, exercise and history, history and exercise, would come up. Occasionally, I'd jot a note on a scrap of paper and stuff it into a desk drawer—for instance: "*Freud biography, p. 183—See footnote.*" I had dog-eared a page describing how some of Sigmund Freud's early followers shared a passion for physically demanding forms of exercise, a striking contrast to the long periods of sitting required for psychoanalysis. Karl Abraham was an avid swimmer and mountain climber; Ernest Jones, a figure skater. (Jones even wrote a book on figure skating, *The Elements of Figure Skating*, in addition to his own biography of Freud.) As for Freud, he took long mountain walks. That fit. *Do you choose your form of exercise, or does it choose you?* I thought to myself.

Sometimes the exercise and the exerciser just did not match up in my head. Take Franz Kafka, for instance: "Every night for the past week my neighbor in the adjoining room has come to wrestle with me," he confided to his diary in May 1941. "Apparently he is a student, studies all day and wants some hasty exercise in the evening before he goes to bed. Well, in me he has a good opponent; accidents aside, I perhaps am the stronger and more skillful of the two. He, however, has more endurance."

Well, then.

In the newspaper one day, I came across the famous photo of Albert Einstein on a bike, tore it out, and pinned it above my desk. I'd seen this countless times before but now it was with new eyes. Einstein didn't look like a strapping athlete, but he didn't look like he never exercised either. *Did he bicycle often? How far would he ride? Was the bike his?* I proceeded to go through three books on Einstein in search of answers—all elusive—although I did learn that he liked to sail, which suggested that Einstein knew how to swim.

I made a note of it.

And of this: Leo Tolstoy, who shared with Goethe a "taste for bodily exercise, physical training, and physical enjoyment," in the words of Thomas Mann, would take such long bicycle rides—twenty miles or more, even at age sixty—that his wife would suffer terrible anxiety.

I suddenly imagined Tolstoy and Einstein competing in a triathlon. *Which man would win?*

Maybe a woman would instead. What did Marie Curie do after discovering polonium? She and Pierre closed up their tiny lab and spent the summer cycling and hiking in southern France. Upon returning, reinvigorated, she made her most important discovery: radium.

Elsewhere, a fragment from the diaries of Andy Warhol seemed to sum up in three sentences an entire bygone era, mirror balls and all: "Went to a gym. They got me on a machine and tipped me upside down with all my pills falling out of my pockets and my hair almost fell off. Then went to disco."

Flashback: Whatever happened to gravity boots anyhow?

Warhol aside, though, I realized as my project took shape that I was less interested in the trends of recent decades. This wouldn't be a book about SoulCycle and CrossFit and other fads, of which I already had first- or secondhand experience. It would be about the deeper history I did *not* know—about connecting my experience of exercise, an immediate bodily *now*, with the wisdom of the past that had faded from living memory. It would be a personal history, not a definitive one.

I started scribbling down thoughts wherever they occurred to me. If I didn't have a notebook with me, anything sufficed. I made a mess of notes on a paper placemat at a neighborhood restaurant with Oliver one night. The place is closed now, but I still have wine- and food-stained highlights from our conversation:

Can exercise be disembedded from skill? Is exercise itself a skill or is it a means for attaining a skill, at which point it is no longer exercise but is performance?

It probably sounds more profound after you've shared two pitchers of sangria.

THE WORD *exercise* first came into use in English in the fourteenth century; *to exercise* literally meant "to remove restraint" and was used in reference to farm animals. This gave me a fresh perspective: exercise as unbridled activity, anything goes, as long as it involves movement. Yet the word also came to be linked to internal states, to ways of being. One can exercise caution, prudence, restraint, good taste, good manners, the desire to do good, or for that matter, the desire not to. For every virtue, there is a vice to be exercised just as vigorously. You could design a whole workout based on such a scheme.

Sometimes I'd ask people what they did for exercise and why.

A Bronx-born bartender with the body of Superman promised me he was developing a technique that would revolutionize the fitness business. "Seriously, bro."

"Yeah?" I leaned in.

But it was a secret.

A friend's niece, a plump woman in her fifties, exuberant with health, confided that every morning before taking a shower she blasts music and dances nonstop to the same two songs.

My Russian barber said he plays handball, even in the winter. He and his buddies bring buckets of steaming hot water onto an old court in Queens to keep the balls warm and springy, he explained as he buzz-cut my hair.

Handball—my dad's game; one rarely hears of it anymore. And look at wrestling, I thought—once the definitive Olympic sport, very nearly dropped from competition a few years ago. How sad. Are there certain forms of exercise that are similarly endangered or have already gone extinct—unrecorded, undescribed—like languages that are disappearing? Will that stalwart, the StairMaster, soon be consigned to the junk heap of history, too? The time had come, I gradually realized, for me to consult an expert in such matters.

IT WAS A sultry July afternoon, so hot and sticky that the streets and sidewalks in East Harlem were practically empty. I arrived at the address I had been given at one minute before the appointed time, one o'clock. I mopped my brow with the towel I had taken to carrying with me and pulled open the heavy gold door to the New York Academy of Medicine, the venerable 150-year-old research and advocacy institution. I gave my name to the pleasant-looking young security guard who greeted me.

Arlene Shaner, the Historical Collections Librarian, met me in the marble-floored foyer. She was gracious and soft-spoken and in the vicinity of my age. With her tall, thin, slightly curvilinear frame crowned by a nimbus of pewter gray, she called to mind a dandelion in summer, the kind you make a wish on when you're a kid. We took the elevator to the third floor, and I followed her through several rooms, as grand and high-ceilinged as ballrooms and entirely vacant but for books, and then up a winding stairway. She led me down an empty corridor and paused before a door that bore a small, hand-lettered sign in ochre paint: *Rare Books*.

Ms. Shaner unlocked the door and ushered me into the foyer, where we were greeted by six human skulls atop a card catalog. I immediately experienced a multisensory déjà vu as I took in the sight of thousands of volumes lining the walls of two rooms and the distinctive musty aroma of old books. "I love that smell," I murmured. If I were blind, I would have no trouble making my way around the desks and chairs and up one of the ladders to the most ancient book on the highest shelf, by scent alone.

I chose a carrel near Ms. Shaner's desk and unzipped my bag, at which she, as if suddenly picking up a frequency audible only to librarians, voiced a series of preemptory *no*s: no pens—don't even bring one out of your bag, she told me in the firmest but nicest possible way—no bottled water, no food, no cell phones, no photos without her permission.

I absorbed every word without a blink, glad to obey this twenty-first-century Minerva. Rare Books was her domain, and I felt fortunate to be allowed temporary residence. Although using laptops was allowed, somehow I felt it would be unseemly. I left mine where it was and took out a pencil and steno pad.

I had requested in advance ten books to review—a not entirely arbitrary number, ten being neither so large as to appear avaricious nor so small as to seem unserious. I have done my time in research libraries and know the unspoken rules as well. Ms. Shaner rolled over a library cart with the books I had reserved—mainly works by familiar names in the history of medicine—and provided a pile of paper bookmarks and a foam rubber reading stand before retreating to her desk. As she did so, I felt a flush of excitement— butterflies, I suppose—like a diver on the platform or runner in the blocks: *3, 2, 1* . . . I reached for the Hippocrates (why not start at the start?), and it was only then that I noticed there were eleven books, not ten. I pulled the unfamiliar title from the cart. The book was oversized and protected by a sturdy slipcase the color of sand.

"I took the liberty," Ms. Shaner said from her desk. "I think you'll want to take a look at that."

I slid the book from its case and held it carefully in my hands; it was the weight of a small dumbbell or a large human brain. I allowed it to fall open naturally somewhere in the middle. What burst to life before my eyes was a graphic image of two pairs of naked men whose bodies were twisted and entwined, incredibly kinetic for a woodcut engraving. I could not make out whose limbs were whose. These burly men looked like they were locked either in combat or in a deeply romantic embrace—they were wrestling, in other words. I looked over at Ms. Shaner and mouthed, *This is amazing.*

She mouthed *I know*, in return.

We were not even whispering, though no one else was there.

Inside the front cover I found a small typed note that traced the book's provenance. What I had in my hands was a rare and valuable illustrated edition in pristine condition of *De arte gymnastica* (*The Art of Gymnastics*), dated 1573. The author was Girolamo Mercuriale, a name previously unknown to me.

At the time, I could not have foreseen that this book would send me on an expedition that would cross more than two thousand years, touch down in three continents, and lead me to study dozens of forms of exercise. I would visit sumptuous Italian palaces, Grecian ruins, and gyms of all sorts. And I would find myself face-to-face with rare specimens of antiquarian books held fast in archives (and protected by occasionally intransigent librarians). Books whose physical presence—not just their contents but their bindings and foxings, their *smell*—would suggest answers to my emerging questions about how the arts of exercise were invented, lost, and rediscovered.

I turned to the first page.

IT BEGAN WITH a vision: buildings in ruins, a bare trace of what once was. As Mercuriale gazed, "lost in admiration," at the crumbling remains of the spacious bath complexes and gymnasia built by the Greeks and Romans "for the sole purpose of exercise," he had a sudden, brilliant, inescapable thought: He would "restore this lost art to its pristine splendor and ancient dignity" by producing a treatise on the subject. It would be for exercise what Andreas Vesalius's *De humani corporis fabrica* was for anatomy, an atlas of a lost Greco-Roman art. Why no one else has taken this on, Mercuriale noted, "I dare not say: I know only that this is a task of both maximum utility and enormous labor."

Over the next several years, he holed up in libraries in Rome and consulted works by more than two hundred writers from the classical period and beyond. In doing so, he created a Renaissance version of an ancient Greek guide to health and fitness, with detailed descriptions of exercises going back to the fifth century B.C.

But I didn't yet know any of this.

All I knew as I sat in that empty library on that hot summer day was that I could not read Mercuriale's masterwork. It was in another language. The best I could do as I paged through the book was to make out a word that appeared again and again and again: *exercitatio*—Latin for exercise, if I was not mistaken.

Finding Mercuriale

I have taken as my province to restore to the light the art of exercise,
once so highly esteemed, but now dead and forgotten.

—GIROLAMO MERCURIALE, *DE ARTE GYMNASTICA*, 1573

I began to spend spare afternoons in the stacks at the Academy of
Medicine, trading the induced fever of the gym—with its
pounding music and sweating, flushed inhabitants—for the silence
and stasis of the library, with its moist, haunted air and fragile
volumes. The spaces had two forms of muskiness in common, but
not much else.

Ms. Shaner and I had a routine: I placed half a dozen books on
reserve early in the week. She met me in the foyer. We took the
elevator to floor 3. We made the walk to the Rare Books room.
There was a certain formality to all of this that pleased me. I was
given no special access, though I certainly knew my way through the
maze. Like any student, scholar, or medical professional who
consulted her, I had to follow protocol, indeed follow her lead. This
was out of respect for the books, for the institution of a library that

they represent, but also for their all-knowing custodian, Ms. Shaner herself.

It was she who introduced me to the Sophist of athletics, Philostratus; to the German Friedrich Ludwig Jahn and his fellow nationalist gymnastics evangelists; and to Harriet Beecher Stowe's sister, Catharine, the Jane Fonda of the mid-nineteenth century. These were all fascinating figures, with great stories behind them, but I longed to know what Mercuriale had to say. If only I had studied Latin in school, I couldn't help feeling, but even this would not have gotten me very far—Mercuriale wrote in an ornate form of medieval Latin that only specialists can translate today.

Intriguingly, I did hear bits and pieces about him secondhand, as it were. In a lengthy treatise published in 1705, I found the Englishman Francis Fuller the Younger repeatedly citing Hieronymous Mercurialis (the Latin spelling for his name) as a source. Fuller recounted how he employed the Italian physician's exercise regimen to cure himself of debilitating hypochondriasis, a condition brought on by a severe case of itch. He was a man converted:

> One might think that violent perspiration would impoverish the blood, but it is quite contrary, just as in Hot Climates, tho' People Sweat profusely, yet they are rather the more Brisk and Lively for it. And thus Moderate Exercise, by Augmenting the Natural Heat of the Body, will enrich the fluids.

Another Englishman, Richard Mulcaster, was a contemporary of Mercuriale's and headmaster at Merchant Taylors' School (the largest in the country at the time). In his 1581 book on education, *Positions*, Mulcaster advocated incorporating exercise into school curricula—PE classes, essentially. For a resource on the subject, Mulcaster noted: "I know not any comparable to Hieronymous Mercurialis, a verie learned Italian Physician now in our time, which hath taken great paines to sift out of all writers, what so euer concerneth the whole Gymnasticall and exercising argument, whose aduice in this question I haue my selfe much vsed, where he did fit my purpose."

Indeed, it seemed that a good deal of *Positions* was based on Mercuriale's *De arte gymnastica*. How did Mulcaster happen to come upon it? He was in the inner circle of Queen Elizabeth and was apparently acquainted with Shakespeare, who, it has been said, modeled the schoolmaster in *Love's Labor's Lost* after him. Suddenly, the world of the late sixteenth century seemed very small. Could Shakespeare have known of Mercuriale's work as well?

Oddly, the two bore a certain resemblance to each other, if only judging by a portrait engraving I found of Mercuriale. He was bearded and balding and had a bulbous brow, as if to indicate how very great his intelligence was. As for details on the man himself, this much I knew: Girolamo Mercuriale was born in Forli, Italy, the central town in what is now the Romagna region, on September 30, 1530. The son of a doctor, he took a degree in medicine and philosophy from the University of Venice, following studies at home and at the University of Padua. (Padua is where Vesalius had taught anatomy and created his masterpiece, published in 1543, although he was no longer at the university by the time Mercuriale arrived.) Even before graduating, Mercuriale had begun to make a name for himself as a scholar and a medical authority unafraid to challenge the status quo. At just twenty-two, not yet a parent himself, he wrote a treatise on child rearing, titled *Nomothelasmus*, in which he made a case against the use of wet nurses, customary at the time, and in favor of breastfeeding by the mother, which he felt was healthier for a child.

Mercuriale settled down to practice medicine back in his native city. As a physician, he would have attended to the concerns, complaints, maladies, and minor injuries of his patients in a manner not unlike that of a small-town general practitioner today, with one gigantic exception. The practice of medicine at the time still rested on an unscientific premise: the ancient Hippocratic theory of the four humors. Humoral theory held that four internal fluids, or humors—blood, phlegm, yellow bile, and black bile—determined a person's state of health. When one or more of these fluids was over-abundant or insufficient, the body's inner scales tipped and illness resulted, leaving one in a state of "distemper." Treatment, therefore, involved bringing the humors back into balance through such means as bloodletting, purging, fasting, sweating, inducing urination, and administering enemas. That such remedies may have caused as much harm as good seems obvious only in retrospect (although it was the philosopher Francis Bacon who said at the time, "The remedy is often worse than the disease," presumably out of personal experi-ence). During the period Mercuriale was practicing, Vesalian anatomy was still far too new to have made an impact on traditional medicine: William Harvey's discovery of the circulation of the blood by the beat of the heart was sixty years away; and a full under-standing of infectious disease would not coalesce until the nine-teenth century.

Little is known about Mercuriale's day-to-day life during this early phase of his career; however, one can make inferences about his general demeanor. If Mercuriale was mercurial in any way, it was apparently in name alone; he seems to have been a man of even temper, of sanguine rather than bilious or choleric humor. Presumably it was this very quality, together with his keen intellect and scholarly bearing, that earned the regard of the townspeople in Forli, who nominated him to travel on a diplomatic trip to Rome in 1562. There he met Cardinal Alessandro Farnese, a scion of the wealthy and powerful Farnese family and a grandson of the late Pope Paul III. (Yes, grandson—it was not required for a pope to have been celibate at that time.) Farnese was apparently so impressed that he invited Mercuriale to join his household as his personal physician. It was in this position that Mercuriale gained access to the Vatican Library as well as to the Farnese family's extraordinary private library and began to work on the *Gymnastica*, which was but one of a number of books he would write in his long lifetime. He died in Forli at age seventy-six. The last edition of the *Gymnastica* was published in the seventeenth century.

Or so I thought. But then one day, Ms. Shaner referred me to a rare books librarian in Austin, Texas, who informed me of an Italian edition of the *Gymnastica* produced in 1996 by a fine arts publisher in Florence, Italy. It contained a complete English translation, the first such ever done; however, it was out of print and not available in any bookstore or library in New York City, or from online booksellers. I paid what was to me an extravagant sum to buy a remaining copy directly from the Italian publisher and, with this in hand, tracked down the translator. Almost exactly one year after I had first learned of Mercuriale's book, I made a trip to London for no reason other than to meet this person. We agreed to a place and a time, the Wellcome Library for the History of Medicine on the first Monday in July at eleven A.M.

I confirmed the details before leaving New York and, in reply, received a charming email with the following instructions:

> Dear Mr. Hayes,
> I suggest you sit in the periodicals section in the far bay, with the Journals S-Z.
> I'll find you there.
>
> See you, Vivian

I ARRIVED AT the library an hour early, knowing from previous visits that the security protocol there was akin to an airport's— understandable, given the irreplaceable manuscripts housed within.

I found my way to the appointed spot and began acquainting myself with the journal of the Zoological Society of India. There were no library patrons even remotely nearby, which I figured must be why I was instructed to sit there, of all places.

At the stroke of eleven o'clock, Dr. Vivian Nutton sailed in, a tall man in his late sixties with the aspect of a majestic bird, trench coat billowing, beak first. A former Cambridge don, now director of the medical history program at University College London, Dr. Nutton was one of the world's foremost experts on ancient medicine and its practitioners. He had written more than a dozen scholarly books, including definitive works on Galen, and hundreds of academic papers.

Before he had even taken a seat, the first question came—not from me, but him: "So, what's your interest in Mercuriale?" It was delivered with a friendly grin but also with an appraising eye and an unmistakable briskness. I was not through security just yet.

"Curiosity—pure and simple." I explained that I wanted to learn everything I possibly could about Mercuriale—as I tried to learn everything I possibly could about the history of exercise. "And yours, Dr. Nutton?"

I found myself unable to call him Vivian.

He told me that he first encountered Mercuriale about forty years earlier, when he was a fellow at Cambridge and gave a paper on ancient medicine in the Renaissance. "Mercuriale was one of the great scholars, one of the great medics, of the sixteenth century." Although little known today outside academic circles, he was a major figure at the time, one of about half a dozen "big names" who were "primed to reinvent the world of the past because they thought what went before was better." Just as classical art and philosophy were considered the epitome of humankind's achievement in the new spirit of humanism, so too with medicine. "This is the Renaissance, after all."

Dr. Nutton spoke in the clear, ringing cadences of an instructor accustomed to large lecture halls—never mind that we were in a library—and precisely slowly enough that I could take notes without missing a word. I felt as if I were the sole student in an impromptu master class, seated in the front row.

He explained that the *Gymnastica* was written first and foremost with one reader in mind: Cardinal Farnese, to whom the book's first edition was dedicated. Although Mercuriale undoubtedly did his duty as personal physician, he had been given the equivalent of a MacArthur Foundation "genius" grant: the freedom to pursue his intellectual interests at leisure—*otium*, in Latin—while contributing to the larger cultural interest in all things antiquarian, of which Farnese himself was an avid collector. The cardinal remained the dedicatee for the first edition alone, though. By the time Mercuriale had revised the book, adding illustrations and additional material for the 1573 edition (the one I'd first seen at the library), he had received what was perhaps the ultimate promotion. Thanks partly to the success of the *Gymnastica*, he had become personal physician to the Holy Roman Emperor, Maximilian II. There was no question what had to be done: The book would be rededicated, which required some authorial gymnastics on his part.

Dr. Nutton took up my copy of his translation, turned to the opening pages, handed it over to me, then sat back with an amused smile.

The dedication was addressed to "THE MOST INVINCIBLE EMPEROR MAXIMILIAN II":

> What was produced by me with great exertion and application of the mind has met, as I have learned from many quarters, with a not unfavourable reception, if I may say so. This was the reason that impelled me to take up again in recent months this treatise. I have no fear that, since second thoughts are usually better than first, it will fail to appear even more acceptable and

give even greater pleasure. This is why I have not hesitated to do what I dared not do before and dedicate it to your Majesty, as proof of my diligence towards you, since all are agreed that, should a patron be needed for the rebirth of gymnastics, none better could be found than you.

I couldn't help but chuckle. "Remarkable: at once self-effacing, immodest, and obsequious. I gather Mercuriale was an ambitious man."

"Of course, but who wouldn't be?" Dr. Nutton observed. "It's as if you had a nobody who came from Bloomington, Indiana, and ended up as the leading dietetic guru in New York."

"Somebody's got to do it."

"Precisely."

Even so, Mercuriale was not a Renaissance-era Andrew Weil, or Dr. Oz, one whose personality or personal story is central to the book's narrative. Mercuriale wrote nothing about his own exercise or diet regimens. To do so would have been considered not so much improper—though it could have been viewed this way—as irrelevant. "What he is doing is trying to lay down universal principles," to write a medical encyclopedia on the topic, Dr. Nutton explained. That said, "He's clearly advocating exercise, and he must in some sense have been interested in all of it."

This was a far more radical proposition than it may seem now. Exercise and athletic prowess were not considered of any real importance at the time, if they were considered at all. The whole culture of exercise and athletics, as epitomized by the Olympic Games, had been essentially snuffed out with the rise of Christianity more than twelve hundred years before. Constantine the Great, the first Christian Roman emperor, formally banned gladiatorial contests in A.D. 325, and some seventy years later, Theodosius I brought the Olympic Games to an end completely. This wasn't simply because exercise and athletics were antithetical to the tenets of Christianity but instead because athletic competition was linked to pagan rituals (such as blood sacrifices of animals) and dedicated to the pantheon of Greek and Roman gods. Cathedrals replaced gymnasiums as sacred sites; it was the holy spirit—the soul—that was now to be glorified, not the body. Not that this happened overnight or with a single decree. But certainly within a few hundred years, the notion of exercise for the sake of exercise was considered indecent. And by the time Mercuriale took the subject on a thousand years later, the art of exercise was, as he put it, "now extinct."

While it's true, Dr. Nutton pointed out, that Mercuriale's work wasn't the very first printed book on exercise—that credit goes to an obscure Spanish physician, Christobal Mendez, whose slight *Book of Bodily Exercise* was published in 1553—*De arte gymnastica* was the far more substantial, comprehensive, and prodigiously researched of the two (there's no evidence that Mercuriale even knew about Mendez's short book).

In the *Gymnastica*, Mercuriale made the case for exercise almost as a defense attorney might, rather than a doctor—logically, carefully, diplomatically. It is composed of six books, or parts, each of which is meant to build on its predecessor. Individual chapters cover walking, running, swimming, jumping, boxing, wrestling, and many more, including forms of exercise that I had never considered before—laughter, crying, and holding one's breath, for instance. His narrative and rhetorical strategy is to make a statement, present evidence, and then call on ancient writers to bolster his argument, pro or con. Mercuriale's primary witness throughout is the Greek-born physician Galen of the second century, whom he cites forty-five times within the first hundred pages alone. This is not surprising. The teachings of Galen had formed the basis of medical education and thought in the West for fourteen centuries.

I asked Dr. Nutton about himself: Did translating the *Gymnastica* have an impact on his own exercise routine? He demurred. "I was reasonably sporting in my youth; I used to play squash, cricket, tennis, and now I go down to the gym two or three times a week," so Mercuriale can't be given credit for keeping him in shape at his age. In any case, Dr. Nutton added, his major physical activity is one that Mercuriale doesn't even mention. "I ring church bells—"

"Church? Bells?"

He nodded. "In the village where I live. Wednesday nights, sometimes Monday night, some Saturdays, Sunday mornings, of course. It's very physical: You pull on a rope."

This part I could imagine—engagement of the lats, biceps, hand muscles—a tug-of-war with God. But the bell? What were we talking about here—*The Hunchback of Notre-Dame* or *The Sound of Music*?

"The ones we have in the village are about six hundred pounds. The heaviest I've rung is forty-some hundred weight."

I made a mental note to seek out a church bell to ring in New York.

The version of the *Gymnastica* that Dr. Nutton translated was the last of five editions that Mercuriale completed—like his contemporary, the French essayist Montaigne, he tinkered with and added to his work—so presumably his publisher was making enough of a profit to warrant going to the trouble to reissue it. Yet it didn't inspire a whole spate of copycat exercise books in the sixteenth and seventeenth centuries, which is curious, especially since "how-to," medical advice, and comportment guides had come into vogue, as the printed book—then roughly in its hundredth year—flourished. It would be another three centuries before the subject of exercise was taken up again with such rigor and passion.

I didn't get it, I had to admit. Why didn't Mercuriale's book make more of an impact? It's not as if it were lost to history.

Dr. Nutton started to say something, then paused, clearly weighing his words. "I think it's a big book," he said finally.

If anyone had earned the right to say so, it was the translator. I glanced at the fat volume sitting between us. "If only it had been shorter, in other words?"

He put it more diplomatically: "I think people *knew* it. It's clearly one of the books you like to have on your shelves—"

"—like the Bible or *Infinite Jest*."

His eyes narrowed, as if he didn't see the connection.

"But do you *read* it?" I said.

"Does one?" the translator corrected.

Gym Rats

We in no way dispute that exercise . . . can sometimes be hard and,
when it is being performed, unpleasant. But good health is
not incompatible with some discomfort.

—GIROLAMO MERCURIALE, *DE ARTE GYMNASTICA*, 1573

I was now determined to learn something new each time I exercised—to find the art in the sweat, so to speak, Mercuriale style. I returned to my hotel, changed out of my suit, and went in search of the gym on the lower level. Correction: Fitness Center, it was called. Either way, if Mercuriale were here by some miracle, he would think there must be a mistake. In his mind, "A gymnasium was a public place built in a separate area of the city," as it was in Athens. "The capacity of these places was so large, their area so great in extent, that it was possible to carry out without any hindrance innumerable exercises of diverse types, of both body and mind." Plato and Aristotle, he pointed out, attracted crowds at gymnasia to discuss philosophy.

Alas.

What I find in the basement of my hotel is a room not much larger than mine upstairs. To my immediate left is a truncated version of a universal gym, with cables for performing pull-downs, triceps extensions, biceps curls, and such. To my right: a treadmill, circa 1990. A rowing machine and a selection of lightweight dumb-bells are tucked into the far corners of the room.

There are no philosophers present.

There is only me—reflected infinitely in the mirrors lining two walls of the room—and a giant red Bosu ball for company. I say "Hello" and give it a shove. I grab a rubber mat and begin the warm-up I do to start every workout, a mix of things I've picked up over the years from trainers and physical therapists or by watching other gym rats. I firmly believe that the gym is one place where copying is never cheating, and I regularly steal from others. I always start with a standing hamstring and calf stretch—hands against a wall, one leg flexed, the other extended back, heel down on the floor, hold for thirty seconds, then switch legs. If there's a flight of stairs nearby, I run up and down them eight or ten times—there's hardly a better, quicker full-body warm-up.

I move on to shoulders and chest: I start by flapping my arms like an alarmed pelican, then lower them near my hips and do the same. Arms raised laterally and elbows bent, I position myself in a corner and push my chest forward as far as I can—as if my chest were trying to kiss the corner; this gets back muscles engaged as well. Since I'm still standing, I loosen my neck—rotate it, side to side, every which way, as if my head were doing a belly dance—and do a bunch of shoulder shrugs and rotations. Down on the mat, I do a V stretch—more hamstrings, which are always tight; lie on my back, pull my knees in one at a time, stretch the hips and glutes; and finally, with a knee pushing hard against the ankle on the opposite leg to pull it toward the chest, stretch the piriformis, a pear-shaped muscle deep within the thigh. I flip over—knees tucked, head burrowed between arms outspread—and stretch my back muscles and shoulders, a classic yoga "child's pose." This whole routine takes seven to ten minutes.

Some say I should not do any of this. Recent scientific research shows that stretching before working out actually reduces one's strength and power by expending energy in muscle tissue. I don't care. I'm not training to be a competitive power lifter. Stretching before working out is what I am used to; it's part of my routine; and what's more, it feels good to me. That's reason enough. Stretching warms you up psychologically, if not anatomically. Mercuriale sides with me: "Everyone should begin with a relaxed and gentle exercise," he writes, "increasing its intensity gradually."

Warming up in such a way fell into the first of three distinct categories of exercise in Mercuriale's eyes: preliminary, simple (the main workout), and terminal (equivalent to a cooldown). The preliminary stage was more specific than one might expect today. "First," Mercuriale writes, "clean the body, comb the hair, wash the hands and face, [and] dress appropriately." Mercuriale recommends clothes that do not obstruct movement but do protect against winds and heat. In saying so, the doctor departs emphatically and unapologetically from ancient tradition, for the very word that appears in the title of his book, *gymnastics*, comes from the Greek term for "exercising in the nude," the standard practice in ancient Greece for hundreds of years.

Missing from Mercuriale's tome is any mention of specific exercises for abdominal muscles—crunches, sit-ups, and such. The same is true of works by Galen and others who had written about exercise in antiquity. This is not because a paunch was especially prized (as it would be during other periods, when a big stomach was, for men, suggestive of power, wealth, and robust health, and for women, of both motherhood and luscious sensuality). Nor is it because the Greeks and Romans failed to appreciate the aesthetics of well-defined abdominal muscles; one has only to look at the six-packs chiseled into ancient statuary and the painted vases depicting athletes with lean, well-defined waists. Instead, participating daily in strenuous athletic activities and doing manual labor likely developed these powerful trunk muscles, no further effort required.

I, on the other hand, spending most days at a desk, can only aspire to the obliques of a discus thrower, the rippling rectus abdominis of a young wrestler. My strategy is to do any and every variation of sit-ups I can think of, in every possible direction, and at different speeds: fast, glacially slow, long holds, both on and off the giant Bosu ball. If I'm at a gym with abdominal machines, I use them, too. But one thing I never do is count. First of all, I always lose count when I'm doing sit-ups. But more, I think that counting the number of sit-ups creates a false sense of achievement. The goal should not be to reach one hundred but to exercise the abdominal muscles to exhaustion—all of them. There are two levels of muscle below those seen near the surface (if one is so lean or so genetically blessed). My rule of thumb is this: An abs workout is not an abs workout unless one breaks out in a sweat.

I take a seat on the rowing machine, not a cardio device that I often use. To distract myself from the absurdity of enacting rowing without a boat, body of water, or place to go, I focus purely on technique. Correcting my posture: back straight, shoulders down. Feeling the spring in my legs and arms. Rhomboid muscles retracting, pulling back my shoulder blades, the scapulae; I picture the wings of a predatory bird opening. I watch the cable snap back and forth. Music is playing in my ears, and the cable seems to mimic the rhythm. I row for ten minutes, and though there is no heart monitor, I can tell that my heart is beating at a good pace—110 beats per minute or so—and I am breathing at least twice as rapidly as usual. I have now officially met Mercuriale's definition of exercising:

> Strictly speaking, exercise is a physical movement that is vigorous and spontaneous, which involves a change in

breathing pattern, and is undertaken with the aim of keeping healthy or building up a sound constitution.

In its concision and clarity, his definition could serve perfectly well today. Mercuriale borrowed from Galen, who had defined exercise fourteen hundred years earlier as "vigorous movement" that causes breathing to increase, but he added an important distinction with his final clause about the "aim" of exercise. Mercuriale felt that *intention* is the critical factor separating exercise from work and other forms of movement. Take digging, for example: "If its purpose is to cultivate the soil and grow fruit, then undoubtedly it should be called work and labor; but if its aim is health then it should be called exercise." So, too, with rowing: If the sole purpose is to get across a lake, then rowing is not exercise per se but a form of transportation.

This notion of *intention* is also useful in distinguishing exercise from sports. Virtually by definition, sports imply competition, rules to play by, and, whether we are talking about team or individual sports, the declaration of a "winner" and a "loser." Of course, you can get exercise when playing basketball or tennis or even golf (some say), but exercise is secondary to the actual intention of engaging in sports, which is to compete against others in a game of some kind and, hopefully, to trounce your opponent.

AS I MOVE toward the weight machine, I am finding it hard to decide if this pocket-sized gym with its strange contraptions would please or displease the doctor from Forli. Would Mercuriale appreciate that there is a gymnasium, small as it may be, or would he be appalled by its size and absence of amenities? In ancient Greece and in the early Roman Empire, there was at least one gymnasium in every town. The gymnasium was as much a part of culture and society as a theater and marketplace—albeit a place for men and boys of the upper classes alone. Women were not permitted into gymnasia— even just to watch. While it's true that Plato says in the *Laws* that "women, both young and old, should exercise . . . together with the men," *should* does not mean they could or did but suggests an ideal, one that, in reality, didn't occur broadly until the nineteenth century. Mercuriale, neither advocating nor opposing the notion of women exercising in gyms, neatly sidesteps the issue: "It is not the place to investigate here."

Gyms were generally official buildings, owned by the city, and with dedicated staff, including trainers and the ancient equivalent of "towel boys." Day-to-day administration was the responsibility of a general manager called the *gymnasiarch*. Private gymnasia existed, too, and for these, records confirm, visitors paid fees just as one does today—they were gym members, essentially. By the sixteenth century, in Mercuriale's Italy, the only gymnasia left were in shambles—half-buried relics of major buildings, such as the Baths of Caracalla.

Mercuriale had fixed, even grandiose, ideas about what a gymnasium is, how one should be designed and built, based on the text of the Roman architect Marcus Vitruvius. His ten-volume work, *De architectura* (*On Architecture*, ca. 25 B.C.), the only surviving major book on classical architecture, provides specific design details on everything from aqueducts and central heating to the construction of prisons and theaters, as well as the machinery and materials that were used. In the fifth volume, chapter 11, he describes the "rules" for a proper *palestra*, the name given by the Greeks to a large athletic facility devoted to wrestling and with spaces for exercising, viewing, and bathing. (The ancient Greek word for "gym rat"—yes, they had them, too—literally translates as "palestra addict.")

Vitruvius specifies a large central courtyard, four hundred meters square (the same length as a standard running track today) to serve as the main area for exercise. This must be bordered on three sides by single porticoes designed for walking, within which are "seated halls" where philosophers, rhetoricians, "and others who delight in study may sit and dispute." The fourth side is a double portico with additional seating and a roof to keep walkers dry on rainy days. Within the double portico, a series of rooms is required: an oiling room, where one is anointed with scented olive oils before exercising in the nude; a "powdering room," where finely ground dust is applied over oiled skin, whether to protect it from the sun or to make it less slippery, more tactile; and finally a series of bathing rooms—cold and hot baths, sauna, and a "vaulted sweating room." On the opposite side of the palestra is a sunken walking path about twelve feet wide. "Thus," Vitruvius writes, "those who in their clothing walk round the paths, will not be incommoded by the anointed wrestlers who are practicing." Behind this whole complex is a stadium, large enough "that a great number of people may commodiously behold" athletes contending in competition.

Mercuriale included a blueprint for just such a Vitruvian gymnasium in the first edition of his book. Though the gym of his dreams was idealized, however, the bodies he envisioned exercising there were not. He would not approve of the hypertrophied muscles of bodybuilders we see today, male and female alike. "Strength is very different from good health," Mercuriale emphasizes, "[Those who] were over-concerned with beefing up their bodies and gaining greater strength . . . produced minds and senses that were dull, torpid, and slow." Even to aspire to such a body would be a "perversion" of the art of gymnastics. One didn't exercise to enhance one's beauty. That's pure vanity. One exercised to prevent illness and preserve health. He writes, "Those who exercise moderately and appropriately can lead a healthy life that does not depend on any drugs, but those who do so without proper care are racked by perpetual ill health, and require constant medication."

Mercuriale was, in this way, both ahead of his time—anticipating the modern concept of preventive medicine, with its focus on diet, exercise, and behavioral modification—and upholding ancient practices. A wrestler-turned-physician named Herodicus, who lived in Athens in the fifth century B.C., is credited with developing the idea, but it was his student, Hippocrates, who fully articulated the tenets of exercise as medicine. "Eating alone will not keep a man well; he must also take exercise," Hippocrates stated. "For food and exercise, while possessing opposite qualities, yet work together to produce health."

Hippocrates wrote two treatises on healthful living, *Regimen in Health* and *Regimen*, covering diet, exercise, rest, bathing, and other matters of hygiene. (The titular word comes from the Latin *regere*— to rule or govern; hence, a regimen provides rules by which one should live.) He emphasized that one must pay careful attention "to proportion exercise to bulk of food, to the constitution of the patient, to the age of the individual," and so on; in other words, a regimen must be customized to the person and, by definition, incorporated into daily life. It is from these ancient beginnings, it's no stretch to say, that our modern notion of a workout plan derives.

I AM NOTHING if not loyal to my back. Here—not with chest, arms, or legs—is where my weight training workouts always start. Monday is back; back is Monday; no exceptions: this has long been my practice. Even so, I don't lift nearly as heavily as I once did. I can't. A few years ago, I tore a rotator cuff tendon—one of the four small muscles that stabilize the shoulder—as a result of years of weightlifting (on top of the normal deterioration that comes with age). It wasn't serious enough to require surgery, but it was extremely painful and kept me out of the gym for months—I could not raise my arms above chest level—while I did twice-weekly physical therapy.

Plato could have warned me. In the *Republic* he advises "temperance" in physical training, likening it to learning music and poetry.

Keep it "simple and flexible"; as in all things, don't overdo. Follow this course, and you will remain "independent of medicine in all but extreme cases."

He spoke from personal experience. Plato was an athlete, particularly skilled as a wrestler. His given name was Aristocles, after his grandfather, but the coach under whom he trained is said to have called him "Plato"—from the Greek for broad, *platon*, on account of his broad-shouldered frame. It stuck. So good a wrestler was Plato that he reportedly competed at the Isthmian Games (comparable to the Olympics, one of four major athletic festivals in the Greek world), and continued wrestling into adulthood. Ensconced at the Academy, one of Athens's largest gymnasia, he spoke strongly on behalf of the virtues of exercise and physical education. He felt that one should balance physical training with "cultivating the mind," exercising "the intellect in study." The goal "is to bring the two elements into tune with one another by adjusting the tension of each to the right pitch."

Equal parts thought and sweat, in other words.

As one can see most obviously in gifted athletes and performers, the body itself can be a source of knowledge—coordination, grace, agility, stamina, skill—both intuitive and learned. Indeed, there are a rare few who might be called Einsteins of the body—geniuses at inventing, expressing, and employing movement. Is that not what the choreographer Mark Morris is? Or Serena Williams?

The contemporary philosopher (and self-admitted sports nut) Colin McGinn points out that physical education should be a lifelong pursuit. "We like our minds to be knowledgeable, well-stocked with information; we should also want our bodies to be similarly endowed," he writes in his book *Sport*. "The erudite body is a good body to have."

Of course, there is the risk of taking things too far. Again, from the *Republic*: "Have you noticed how lifelong devotion to physical exercise, to the exclusion of anything else, produces a certain type of mind? Just as neglect of it produces another?" Plato writes, recounting the words of Socrates. "Excessive emphasis on athletics produces an excessively uncivilized type, while a purely literary training leaves men indecently soft."

Even if I'd been sitting at Plato's feet as a younger man, I probably would not have listened. Back then, looking good and getting bigger mattered most. I suppose it was all very Darwinian—puffing myself up to attract a mate. But I was not explicitly conscious of such aims. I liked working out in itself, the pure satisfaction of using full force against a resistance. I sought what Ivan Pavlov—a lover of biking, rowing, and swimming—so beautifully called "muscular gladness."

I do still.

I reach overhead and grasp the wide bar used for lat pull-downs (*lat* being short for latissimus dorsi, the sweep of muscle extending from each armpit to the lower back), perch lightly on the bench, lean forward, and pull the bar down as far as I can. I do this slowly, almost luxuriating in the resistance met, until it touches down at midtrapezius, the triangular muscle covering the center of the back, then let it ease back up until my arms are outstretched. Now, again, a little faster, and again, and again, until I reach ten or twelve. Without resting, I shift positions, leaning back and pulling the bar down in front of me to midchest. I think of this as a reverse bench press, pulling rather than pushing, lats and traps engaged rather than the chest muscles. That I cannot see my back in the act is part of what makes this satisfying; one has to picture the muscles, feel them contracting, rely not on sight but on sensation. I finish the set by changing grips: from wide to close, hands almost touching each other, and pull down over and over until my arms and back are exhausted. I rest for a moment. I up the weight by ten.

No Athlete

It is not a mind, it is not a body that we are training;
it is a man, and he ought not to be divided into two parts.

—MICHEL MONTAIGNE (1533–1592)

I was not an athlete as a kid—I didn't do team or school sports—but I was athletic enough that, had I been confident enough, I could have been. I was raised by a father who had been a West Point cadet and fought in Korea. He was a paratrooper, who, even after being blinded in one eye from a combat injury, continued to make jumps, night jumps into enemy territory, he told me. I wonder now what gave him the biggest rush: leaping from the plane, floating through the sky, or crashing to earth and springing back up again? Looking back, I suppose you could say that he lived his whole life in this way and that I have taken after him in this regard.

As exercise was built into his training for being a soldier, so, too, exercise was built into the training he gave me, his only son, in being a man. He taught me how to swim and snow-ski and ride a bike and play ball. We did running drills down the block. We shadowboxed in the garage. He put me on top of a picnic table and showed me the proper way for a paratrooper to land.

He had retired from the army before my folks were married and, practically sight unseen, bought a Coca-Cola bottling plant in Spokane in 1963. Spokane was known as the hub of the "Inland Empire," the largest city in an area comprising western Montana, northern Idaho, and eastern Washington. As a supplier of soda pop to all the stadiums in the region—the largest being the rather grandly named Spokane Coliseum—he got free admission to every imaginable sporting event. I don't recall now whether my mom and five sisters never wished to go or, more likely, were never invited (he called them "the squaws," only half-kiddingly) and were left at home. All I know is that I was always in the stands with him, Son of the Chief, bearing a bag of popcorn and an Orange Crush and a perpetually abstracted expression. I never quite understood the rules by which things were played. We went to baseball games, hockey games, swim meets, track meets, boat shows, car shows, air shows, the rodeo. Had there been bullfighting in Spokane, Dad and I would have been in the front row.

After church on Sundays, he would take me to the Spokane Athletic Club. I remember everything about those trips: the car ride down Comstock Court to Lincoln Street to Monroe, the getting out of the car, the walking from the parking lot up the stairs to the front desk, the opening of the door to an inner sanctum named "Men."

The Spokane Club had all things athletic under one roof: swimming pool, basketball court, handball and squash courts, jogging track, gymnastics equipment (parallel bars, rings, vault), wrestling mats, stationary bikes, punching bag, boxing ring, weight room, sundeck. It was a modern-day Greek palestra—circa 1970.

Note the name: It was not a gym but a *club*. You could not simply walk in and join but had to be accepted, pass muster, be voted in. You *belonged*. That notion, of belonging, became deeply embedded in me and to this day remains linked, inextricably, to working out, to exercising—albeit with a different understanding now than I had back then.

To be a member of the Spokane Club was also to know implicitly that some of the citizenry was not allowed in. There were no Jewish or Black members at the time, I've been told. Not that there were many Jewish people or Black people in Spokane in any case. The few who did live there all seemed to work at the club, as waitresses and cooks and shoeshine men and janitors. The masseur was an elderly and blind Black gentleman. The club's logo incorporated an Indian chief, but needless to say there were no Spokane Indians at the Spokane Club either (the Spokane Reservation was fifty miles outside town). Women were allowed but tended to be members by virtue of being wives or daughters. That the club's membership, ethos, and unspoken rules reflected, in microcosm, the culture of Spokane itself is obvious to me only in retrospect. At nine or ten, I didn't yet know enough to know, to really know, how segregated a place could be. With one exception: From a young age, I did know at some level that being a boy in my family, especially being the only boy, gave me privileges my sisters did not automatically receive. After all, only I got a bedroom to myself, got new clothes (not hand-me-downs or homemade ones), got to do things my sisters could not do, even if I did not want to do them. I was allowed to be an altar boy at our Catholic church—to literally be on an altar—just as only my dad, not my mom, could be a lector at mass.

The Spokane Club was not unlike the church in this way. It was a men's club, first and foremost, and nowhere more so than in the locker room. Here there was a steam room and a sauna and a whirl-pool bath and seemingly no rules when it came to nakedness, in stark contrast to home, where squaws outnumbered braves three to one, and extreme modesty prevailed. Freshly laundered towels towered high near the showers, yet most men availed themselves only to dry off and then lounged in the buff or their boxers, playing cards, reading the paper, watching the game on a black-and-white television.

On Sundays, my father had a standing handball game with Dr. Parker. I trailed after Dad as he dashed into the locker room to change out of his church clothes. The lockers were stacked three high, row after row after row after row—more than a church has pews, to my eyes—and painted the aqua blue of the bottom of a swimming pool. They were lockers in name only; no one actually locked them. Contained within, not unlike vestments in a sacristy wardrobe, was *gear*—sweaty, smelly gear. Off went the suit and tie, on went the jockstrap, gym shorts, sneakers, T-shirt, sweatshirt, goggles, and gloves. I watched in awe as my father transformed into an athlete.

SPORTING EVENTS DATE back at least to the Bronze Age, when evidence shows that wrestling and boxing matches were staged as entertainment for the king of Crete, but the concept of an *athlete*, as we know it today, comes to us from ancient Greece. Here, athletic competition was born in the Olympic Games, first held in 776 B.C. Actually, make that Olympic *Game*, singular, for in the beginning there was but one—a sprint of roughly two hundred meters. A man named Coroebus was crowned the winner with a wreath of olive leaves. Seventeen Olympiads later, the discus, the javelin, the long jump, and wrestling were added to the competition; boxing and other sports followed soon after. (Although some team sports were played at the time, these were never part of athletic competitions, the emphasis for glory being on the individual.)

Like their counterparts today, Olympic athletes developed the strength, speed, skill, and stamina needed to compete through systematic exercise regimens—lifting, jumping, sparring, throwing, grappling, running. In a sense, this gave fitness training a new meaning, a new identity, and placed exercise on a path toward eventual popularization with the masses. This was a departure from the past. In its earliest incarnation, exercise was meant not for the sake of athletics, much less for health or beauty, but purely as preparation for war—to train and equip soldiers for combat. Women were not included in such military training, except for in one place: Sparta, an independent Greek city-state that emerged around the tenth century B.C. and rose to prominence over the next five hundred years. Spartan society was focused exclusively on warfare, and for this reason women and girls were expected to train alongside men and boys, whether to prepare themselves for combat or to keep in shape for the purpose of bearing healthy male children who would become exceptional warriors.

Women also were not allowed to compete in the Olympic Games except by proxy, so to speak, and in a single event: If wealthy enough, a woman could own a team of horses entered into the chariot races. Reputedly, a team owned by a daughter of the Spartan king, Archidamus—her name was Cyniska—won the event in both 396 and 392 B.C. She was not shy about it. Cyniska erected a statue at Olympia to commemorate her victories, which read in part: "I assert that I am the only woman in all Greece who won this crown." And so it would remain until 1900, when women were first allowed to compete at the Olympics held in Paris, the second such games of the modern era (founded four years earlier by the Frenchman Pierre de Coubertin).

But it wasn't just athletic competition from which women and girls had been barred for centuries. Aside from not being allowed inside gymnasia, they were not encouraged, much less permitted, to exercise in public in any organized fashion throughout antiquity. Women were expected to be "modest, chaste, obedient, and inconspicuous," as historian Betty Spears has written, not to be so indiscreet as to train and tone their bodies or to compete. Some contemporary scholars contest this claim, pointing as evidence, for example, to the so-called "Bikini Girls" mosaic created for a lavish Roman villa around A.D. 320 (now a UNESCO World Heritage Site), in which bikini-clad young women were portrayed running, using weights, hoisting a discus, and so on. But even if this stunning mosaic were a true representation of daily life in the early Roman Empire—and *not* a fantastical image of goddess-like women cavorting and competing in games, as other scholars suggest—it would have depicted a rare exception, one reserved for the daughters and wives of wealthy men. For the vast majority of women, the traditional Greek ideal of excellence applied to the domestic arts, child-rearing, and homemaking, not to achieving the height of athletic performance.

THE GREEK WORD from which *athlete* derives has two forms, a masculine form meaning a contest and a neutral form denoting the contest winner's prize. Hence *athlete* embodies both trophy and feat. The first recorded use of the word is credited to Homer; it appears in an unexpectedly comic set piece in book 8 of *The Odyssey*.

Odysseus, shipwrecked, finds his way to the land of the Phaeacians, where he is given a hero's welcome by the king. A great banquet follows; a dozen sheep, eight boars, and a pair of oxen are slaughtered. The wine flows. All is light. But when a bard takes the floor and begins to sing in the most rapturous voice of the Trojan War, Odysseus is moved to tears. He tries but cannot hide his weeping. The king cuts the minstrel short and calls for a change of mood— "games of every kind"—at which "a press of young champions" comes forth. Their names alone make this scene an utter delight: Topsail, Riptide, Rowhard, Surf-at-the-Beach, and Broadsea, among them—"in looks and build the best of all Phaeacians." They have a footrace, wrestle, jump, box, and throw the discus, and when they are done, one young buck approaches Odysseus and challenges him to a contest.

Odysseus, old enough to be the boy's father but not yet past his prime, begs off. "Pain weighs on my spirit now, not your sports—"

"—Oh, I knew it!" another mocks, cutting him off. "I never took you for someone skilled in games, the kind that real men play throughout the world . . . You're no athlete."

No athlete: It is equivalent to saying he's no man.

Odysseus leaps up, grabs a discus heavier than any that had been used, and, in one commanding throw, silences the whole lot of them. "Now go match *that*, you young pups," he says with a laugh.

Accounts differ as to whether there was a god of athletics in antiquity. Some say Prometheus, who created men and women out of earth and tears; some say Hermes, the indefatigable runner. But after a recent rereading of *The Odyssey*, I have begun to think that this god was actually a goddess, Athena. Near the end of the tale, when bruised and battered Odysseus finally returns to Ithaca, Athena ensures that his wife will still find him physically attractive. She crowns the man with beauty and makes him "taller to all eyes, his build more massive," as if with an instant dose of steroids—"The 4-Hour Body" in a single moment. Odysseus steps from his bath, "glistening like a god."

MY FATHER WAS neither especially tall nor built, but the door to the handball court was extremely small so he had to duck down to enter, turning him into a Gulliver for a split second. I would then hike up a couple of flights of stairs to the spectators' viewing area. Dad and Dr. Parker darted around the bright white court in what appeared to be a precisely choreographed dance, a *pas de dads*, you might say. The handball left sprays of black splotches on the walls, just like skid marks from bikes on our driveway, its reverberant *boing* that of a hugely amplified plunk on a harp. Every now and then, a fly ball: According to the rules of the game, this put it out of play. But I always saw it in the opposite way, as the handball equivalent of a home run. I chased it down and tossed it back.

"Thanks, pal," the answer came.

Whether or not he won, my father emerged from handball games a changed man: drenched and dripping, his black hair slicked back, face red, sweating so profusely that in the cooled air I could see steam rising from his back. This was remarkable yet not extraordinary. During the summer, he'd sometimes take me with him to the racetrack. Before making bets, we'd go down to the stables. He seemed to know everyone there, all the groomers and trainers; it was some time before I realized this wasn't so of every boy's dad. He was comfortable among working men, a milieu not unlike that of a military unit, I suppose, and at the Coke plant he employed dozens— truck drivers, taste testers, auto mechanics, line operators, handymen. Which is not to say he was *one* of them; he acted, whatever the context, like the boss. I remember, though, how even he was silenced and made smaller somehow by the horses that would suddenly appear, just off the track. Here they came, one after the other, so magnificent to behold and also just barely under control, panting furiously, great eyes gaping, nostrils flaring—nostrils as big as my ears—tails rising to shit, reeking of sweat, pissing the piss of ten men. Heat rose in clouds from each horse's haunches. I was transfixed. Was there horse in man, or man in horse? I had no reason to doubt the existence of the centaur.

After handball, we'd go for a swim. This is where my father got really serious about exercise. He had been captain of the swim team at West Point and, had it not been for the war, on a path to the Olympics. His specialty was the butterfly, the most physically demanding of swim strokes. "Like a butterfly" is not how I would ever have described it, though; that sounds too delicate. There was a kind of violence to his stroke, how he created not just ripples but what seemed like a whole tide with his churning arms and lurching body. The whole pool knew he was there—which was the point. I stayed near the shallow end and did somersaults.

Finally, we'd head back to the locker room and sit in the sauna bath. The only way in which it resembled a bath to me was that we were naked under our towels. The atmosphere struck me as spooky, how church-quiet and dim it was in there. Were we supposed to pray? Unlike the men assembled there, some supine, some sitting, I kept my eyes open. Dad had his head back, beads of sweat dripping down his face, neck, hairy chest, pooling around his legs. He looked like he'd dozed off. But no; every couple of minutes, he'd run a hand over his body and flick a palm full of sweat onto the hot sauna rocks. A puff of smoke followed a hiss, like birthday candles right after they're blown out.

THE SWEAT OF athletes was considered a prize commodity in the ancient world. What a waste, you might have thought, had you been me two thousand years earlier, watching my dad toss sweat onto the rocks. After competing or simply exercising, athletes would scrape the accumulated sweat and oil from their bodies and funnel it into small pots with a metal tool created expressly for this purpose, a strigil, shaped like a celery stalk. This presumably funky-smelling mixture, called *gloios*, was considered so precious that some went so far as to take scrapings from the bathhouse walls against which athletes had leaned and left sweat tracings from their bodies.

Ancient Greek and Roman writers such as Dioscorides, Pliny the Elder, and Galen all attested to this practice. Pliny reported that the masters of the gladiatorial schools at one time sold such scrapings for eight hundred sesterces, equivalent to thousands of dollars. Hard as this might be to believe, records of ancient business dealings confirm that Pliny and company were correct.

Gloios provided a significant revenue stream for the Greek gymnasia at which it was sold—a needed supplement to membership fees at private gyms. It was used for medicinal purposes, the belief being that gloios must contain the essence of *arete*—the striving for excellence that defined a great athlete. But athletic sweat wasn't used, as one might guess, to enhance athletic performance. It was used to treat the most uncomfortable maladies on one's most private parts—hemorrhoids and genital warts.

While it is easy to look back and smirk at such practices, one could cite a hundred equally questionable ones today—things we take or try, including trends in exercise, to make us stronger, thinner, leaner, harder, less forgetful, less wrinkled, less weary, more youthful, less sad. I am as guilty as the next person. I would anoint myself with the sweat of an athlete if I thought it might make me a more vigorous man.

NOW AND THEN, my father and I would go to the movies—just the two of us. We wouldn't see things I might have wanted to see, whatever that might be, kids' movies, I guess. He wasn't a dad doing a favor for his boy. We'd see things he wanted to see, movies Mom would probably never go to with him. He liked westerns. Cowboys and Indians. War movies. Sports. *All Quiet on the Western Front. Patton. Cool Hand Luke. Downhill Racer. Jeremiah Johnson. Bullitt. True Grit.*

We never went to the fights, but he did take me to see the classic bout in 1971 between Joe Frazier and Muhammad Ali. A film of it was released just months after the match at Madison Square Garden—not exactly a documentary, but something like a "Wide World of Sports" special made for TV and then shown on big screens. It played at the Fox Theater in downtown Spokane. A onetime event, if I remember right. I was ten.

I can still see and smell the theater lobby—popcorn and soda pop at the concession stand, the sweeping stairway to the balcony, the deep purple velvet curtain pulled aside by an usher, who took the tickets and led us down the aisle by flashlight.

I didn't know much, if anything, about Muhammad Ali and his history then; it is only in looking back that I can appreciate the significance of that fight. Born Cassius Clay Jr., he had changed his name when he embraced Islam shortly after winning the world heavyweight championship in 1964. Citing his religious beliefs, he refused to be conscripted into the military to fight in Vietnam and was subsequently convicted of draft evasion and stripped of his boxing title.

Could there possibly have been a man more unlike my own dad—the staunch, white, Irish Catholic, decorated military man? Yet here he was, as close as he could possibly get to a ringside seat, for one reason: to watch a superior athlete fight to reclaim the title of champion—a twentieth-century gladiatorial match between two Black men.

That this wasn't the usual movie audience was obvious even in the pitch-dark. Wives, daughters, and mothers had been left at home; supper could wait; this was a congregation of men, including fellows who worked at the Spokane Club. Maybe they'd seen the match on TV already and wanted to see it again. Maybe they'd missed it. But this was something you couldn't see on TV anyplace. TVs were small at that time—sixteen inches at most maybe. The theater screen would turn Ali and Frazier, already mythic figures, into giants.

My father leaned over to ask if I could see the picture over the heads of the men in front of us. His breath was the scent of Scotch—how his words, his voice, often smelled.

I nodded. The theater quieted. The fight began.

They went all fifteen rounds. Frazier, in a surprise decision, won. I don't remember exactly how I felt as we filed out of the Fox and went back home. Had I been mesmerized? Horrified? Maybe I was thrilled by the blood, the sweat, the supreme athletic beauty, the dance. All I know for sure is this: Something in me wanted to know what it's like to be in a fight. Almost forty years later, I'd get my chance.

A Boxer's Diary

The ancient weapons were hands, nails, and teeth.

—LUCRETIUS, *ON THE NATURE OF THINGS*, FIRST CENTURY B.C.

Thursday, March 13

I take a deep breath and walk into the Titanium Training Center. It's just five blocks from my apartment in San Francisco. I have passed it hundreds of times before but never had the courage to go in. The acrid smell of sweat is unmistakable. The gym looks nothing like the gyms I have been going to for the past thirty years, and not just because there isn't a single gay man in sight. It is one big, white, cement-floor room lit by fluorescent bulbs, with a full-scale boxing ring, one mirrored wall, four or five punching bags, and absolutely no frills.

Behind the counter is a man of about thirty who has a shaved head and both the aspect and the build of a nightclub bouncer. I say hello and casually inquire about classes.

He starts to explain that there's a cardio kickboxing class on Wednesdays, but I cut him off: "I am not interested in getting fit. I am already fit. I want to learn how to box."

This news does not surprise him. This is a boxing gym, after all.

I look him straight in the eye. "I would need to start at zero. I have never put on a pair of boxing gloves. I have never hit anyone before in my life."

The bruiser behind the counter does not flinch. "I'll teach you," he says. "Boot camp starts Monday. Five days a week, six weeks. Be here at six A.M."

Monday, March 17

I wake at 5:15 and give myself just enough time for a shower and coffee before heading to the boxing gym. It's chilly and still dark. I can see the stars. I listen to one Björk and half of a U2 song on the way, all I have time for. I cannot be late. "If you're late, even on the first day," Ken, the fellow I'd met yesterday, had told me, "you're going in the drink. Rule number one of boot camp. On Friday, down at Brannan and First, anyone who's been late that week"—he motions a dive with his hand—"in the Bay."

I make it with a few minutes to spare, sign in, dump my stuff in a corner and take a quick glance at my fellow recruits, mostly young men but five or six women, too. At six A.M. sharp, Ken barks, "Start jumping!" One by one, we pick up jump ropes from bins in the corners. There is no music. No one speaks. No rah-rah words of welcome. There is only the sound of twenty-five vaguely terrified people jumping rope. I close my eyes, and it sounds like rain on a tin roof.

But Ken wants to hear a storm. "Come on, people!" he yells. "This is not skipping through the park on a Sunday. Faster! You're not little girls here!"

I am quickly gaining a whole new respect for little girls. They make jumping rope look easy.

"Okay, drop the ropes! Hit the deck: fifty push-ups! One, two, three, four—"

I am face-to-face with the dirty floor when it hits me that I have been here before. Years earlier, before this was a boxing gym, it was a used bookstore. My partner, Steve, and I would come here on Sunday afternoons. Every wall was covered floor to ceiling with bookshelves, and there were rolling ladders so you could climb up and reach books on the top shelves.

"—Now twenty-five more—"

Where the boxing ring is now, at the front window, there used to be an open office area filled with desks and tables and chairs, all holding stacks and stacks of books. A cat or two prowled the territory. It was kind of a dump, but the books were cheap and plentiful and the atmosphere quieter than in most libraries—

"—A hundred sit-ups!" Ken yells.

After that, he tells us to take a breather—by which he must mean a breath, because seconds later he orders us out the door and onto the streets, where we do a two-mile run. This is just our warm-up. When we get back to the gym, we have three quarters of an hour more to go—mostly calisthenics. By the time class one of boxing boot camp ends, every joint hurts and I am so drenched in sweat as to feel amphibious.

It is said that people cannot accurately remember the sensation of pain once it's passed. I now think the opposite holds true as well: You cannot imagine it ahead of time either.

Tuesday, March 18

Boxing is so much about the body—*using* the body, feeling the body, every part, drawing out its power, its grace—but in the boxing gym the body is covered up. Skin is not exposed. Paul, who alternates with Ken as a coach, wears tights under his shorts, a long-sleeved shirt, a cap, as do most of the guys in the class. They wear sweatpants and knit caps and hoodies. I felt completely underdressed yesterday in my sleeveless T-shirt and gym shorts. Today I wear a sweatshirt and longer, baggier shorts.

Class begins with Paul showing us how to wrap our hands for sparring. We had been instructed to buy 108-inch wraps. The exactness of this figure—not 100, not 110, but 108—fascinates me. No doubt, this represents the culmination of years of testing this crucial piece of equipment. Mine are red, as if already blood-saturated. The elastic stitched into the cloth is loose, like an Ace bandage used for one too many sprains.

Paul unfurls a roll in a single toss, then starts wrapping his left hand: three times around the palm, three around the wrist, then threading the wrap in between each finger. Finally, the last phase, round and round and round till you reach the knuckles: "This is called covering your mess." Clearly, this is a line he's said before—he pauses to get the laugh—still, it makes him smile. He proceeds next to wrap his right hand, then pulls on a pair of boxing gloves, tightens them—pulling on the Velcro strip with his teeth—and immediately starts demonstrating combinations. It's as if the wraps and gloves have transformed him, conferred some new power. The way he moves! He looks like a hip-hop dancer, grinding into it, gritting his teeth, *feeling* it, hearing some music inside himself.

My completed hand wraps are a mess that never do get covered up, but they will do for now. Paul stands before us and breaks down the classic boxer's stance: feet together, arms at your sides. Next, bring your hands above your head, put them together as if in prayer, then lower your elbows until your fists float in front of your face.

"Pay attention!" he demands as we practice doing this. "Look at the lines of the body—the backs of your forearms should line up with your quads. See?" He demonstrates again. We can tell by the tone of his voice that this is not a small matter, not something to be hurried through or dismissed.

"Notice the lines," he adds in a quieter voice, almost a whisper, "notice the lines." And in the moment he seems less like a boxing coach and more like a kind of anatomy aesthete.

"Now, form a window in front of your face with your hands and look through it. Elbows in! Okay, you're set. Now, go! Break the glass."

From here, we are to jab through the window with our fists—one, two; one, two—*pow*!

I see myself grimacing in the mirror. It helps to think of this as a form of yoga several levels beyond Vinyasa: violent yoga, shall we say.

One, two; one, two—*pow*!

I begin to get the hang of it, the rhythm of it, but not everyone does. At one point, I see Paul coaching a student who's all elbows, no lines—no fists to speak of either. "You're not going to get it in a day, brother," Paul tells him in what I could swear is a kind voice. "It's a language, a whole new language," he says of these moves we are trying to teach ourselves, we apprentices in this ancient tongue.

Wednesday, March 26

There was no boxing ring as such in the sport's earliest incarnations— no raised platform even. An area would be marked off on the dirt ground with a measuring rod. That was it—*let the fight begin*, as in that brutal scene from the *Iliad*, the match between Epeus and Euryalus: "When the two men were ready, they walked out into the center, put up their fists, and began to punch, and the blows fell quickly. There was a terrible cracking of jaws, and the sweat poured down their bodies."

Much of what we know of boxing in its earliest form comes to us not from boxers but from artisans, poets, philosophers, spectators— witnesses. The so-called Boxer vase from the ancient Minoan settle- ment of Hagia Triada, dated circa 1500 B.C., shows a victorious boxer standing over his fallen opponent. Both wear what look like close-fitting helmets, possibly of leather, and their hands are similarly covered with straps of leather.

The early Greek philosopher and writer Philostratus asserted that boxing was "discovered" by the Spartans in roughly the tenth century B.C. The purpose: to gain strength and skill for hand-to-hand combat in war, a criterion that put it in a whole different category from health-oriented exercise. Plato endorsed this form of training, even during times of peace: "If we were in charge of boxers or competitors in similar athletics, would we send them straight into the contest without any prior training or practice?" he observes in the *Laws*. Certainly not. "[We] would be . . . training and practicing all the methods which we intended to use on the day of the real fight, and imitating the real thing as far as possible."

FOR SPARRING, WE are issued head guards and groin guards—the latter, made of soft thick plastic, resembling comically oversized jockstraps for the Michelin Man. We bring our own mouth guards and gloves. But all this padding is deceptive. What I hadn't seriously considered when I signed up for boot camp is that *getting* to hit someone means that someone is also going to hit *me*—hit me back, if not hit me first—and that it will not be painless. As it turns out, I am a champ at this: *POW*!

That, thank you very much, was courtesy of the tall redhead with the icy blue eyes and long, muscular arms. *POW, POW, POW*: as was *that* series of blows—a couple to the forehead, one to the side.

In the moment, I almost expected an apology.

I thought he would stop and ask if I was okay.

He did not. He didn't say anything. Nor did he smile. He just looked at me and—*POW*—popped me again. The hit was to the head. The impact was at the base of the neck. The sensation was not of being scared—that takes moments to register—but of being *threatened*. That's what makes adrenaline flood the bloodstream.

He was doing exactly as he was told: "Suit up—groin guard, head gear, hand wraps, gloves, everything," Paul had instructed first thing that morning, "then pair up and start sparring." I was the one who was not following instructions. I should have been blocking Red's punches, catching them like a baseball, exactly as Paul had demonstrated. But each time Red's glove came shooting out at me, I was too stunned to do anything. The force of the blow!

One might think that defending oneself, blocking hits, would come naturally—instinctively. But of course, another well-proven method is simply to take flight—flee the scene. Staying, literally staying with it, in the fight, is a hard lesson, I was learning.

"Okay, switch it up!" Paul yells.

Now I am with someone else. I don't know who this is. Have I seen him in class before? I can hardly see his face through the oversized headgear. He's Asian, about my height, which makes catching his blows easier, since he's not bearing down on top of me. Still, I'm floundering, so I take charge of the situation. "Let's break it down," I tell him. "You throw the punches and I'll be on defense."

We are essentially doing it in slow motion. This works; I start to find a rhythm and figure out what I am supposed to be doing. Even as I write this sentence, though, I recognize my problem: I was trying to *remember* what to do, *remember* how to block a punch. But there's no *time* for remembering. In that split second, you make yourself vulnerable, leave yourself open to hits. Instead, you just have to *know* it—in your muscles, in your limbs, in your body—and *do* it: Defend yourself. Trust yourself. Fight.

I suppose this is what I am also here to learn: how to dwell less in memory and more in the moment. After all, one cannot live—any more than one can fight—in slow motion. The blows that truly devastate come out of nowhere.

Sunday, April 6

I keep thinking about the bat in the closet. A black baseball bat. Steve kept it in our clothes closet, in the corner, just to the right of the door.

To him, the bat was not a baseball bat; it was a club, a crude weapon, like something Fred Flintstone would carry. He'd had it for years. I remember him saying when we moved in together that he'd gotten the bat while living in Chicago after college. He was mugged late one night while walking home. He was a big guy and wasn't hurt but was badly shaken. After that he wanted to have some kind of weapon, in case anything ever happened—a stranger at the door, a burglar lurking on the fire escape, that kind of thing. He never had to use it, but just knowing it was in the apartment, in the same place—he could have it in his hands, ready to swing, without turning on the closet light or reaching for his glasses—gave him a degree of security. In a larger sense, he, in turn, provided that for me. He was always there. In our apartment, at my side, at the other end of the phone, a presence. And then one day, he wasn't. Here, then not here—vanished, as if into thin air. Like the bookstore that disappeared.

I woke one morning to a great thrashing, as if the San Andreas had finally given way. My first thought was that Steve must be having a nightmare. I tried but couldn't wake him. I called for help, began CPR, EMTs came. I remember how they kept asking me if we'd been doing drugs. The question seemed absurd, laughable. Steve, who had HIV, was so clean living, he never even drank a beer. They got him to the ER. But by then he was gone: a heart attack. It was inexplicable. He was just forty-three and, by all appearances, perfectly fit. There were no signs, no premonitions, the night before.

We'd worked out at the gym, made dinner, watched TV, read in bed, oblivious to how it would end. He had every expectation of waking up the next day and getting things done. I know because he left a to-do list on his desk: *check light socket, get batteries, buy thread*, and so on. I knew exactly what he meant: . . . *in hall*, . . . *for flashlight in car*, . . . *to repair chair*.

In the weeks that followed, I was able to check off every item on the list. Then I sat down and made one for myself—a list of things I had long wanted to do but hadn't gotten to yet. I did the easy ones first. I went to Paris. I got a camera and started taking pictures. I got a tattoo—and then another, and another, and another, enough ink, in fact, for a whole slew of lists. Finally, a year and a half later, I worked up the nerve to take on one of the tougher challenges I had given myself: *learn to box*.

Monday, April 7

Every day of boxing boot camp starts with at least a half hour of calisthenics—jumping rope, push-ups, sit-ups, jumping jacks, running in place, and then often a run outdoors. Today, before the sun had risen, we were outside the gym, sprinting up the hills. One morning we ran all the way from Glen Park to Twin Peaks—an uphill climb of three and a half miles in the cold and fog that I hope never to do again for the rest of my life. The ancient Roman historian Vegetius once observed that running is the best training for war; I can now see how it would make you want to kill someone.

Last Tuesday, we ran as a group down to Civic Center, where we spent an hour running laps around the entire plaza, and sprinting, doing drills, and sparring on the grass. This was hard work physically but I loved being outside—in the cold, in the predawn darkness, and in front of City Hall, as if we were a bunch of Rocky wannabes. I was pretty good at the drills. Not great—my sprinting skills prompted coaching from Ken—"Pump your arms, Billy! You're not movin' 'em! Fucking pump 'em!" But I was able to cross every finish line, run my laps, and do the endless squats, jumping jacks, and crunches without puking or, like some others, giving up.

Back in the boxing gym, I still struggle. On defense, I flinch or, just as ineffective, jump the gun, blocking punches before they come. As usual, I overthink: *Okay, now which hand blocks? Right? Left?* In the moment, I forget everything I have learned during drills. This doesn't escape Paul's notice. He's on top of me, telling me what I'm doing wrong, showing me how to do it right, and overall, getting frustrated. Truth is, he's getting frustrated with everyone.

In the midst of drills today, he tells us all to take off our gear, just leave wraps on. We face the mirror and do nothing but practice the most basic offensive move, the one-two punch. This is the foundation for every move in boxing. Here's how it breaks down: jab with your left as you step forward, then, when your right foot is planted, jab with your right, pivoting as you do so. Simple, right? One would think so. I certainly would. I know how to do this, but don't make the mind-body connection. I forget to step forward when I jab with my left. Or, I jab with my right before—

"Billy! Goddammit! You gotta plant your right foot before you pivot!" I almost feel sorry for Paul, he looks so disgusted. "How many times do I have to tell you?"

But that's the thing: The *telling* doesn't do it, doesn't help, doesn't trick my body into instantly doing it correctly.

Friday, April 11

Do I catch on less quickly because I am older, my memory less limber, or for a host of other reasons? After all, a muscle memory is not made in the muscle itself but in the brain, essentially through the same pathways along which one learns motor activities as a child— crawling, walking, climbing—as well as "procedural memories," like driving a car. Here, the drills, the sparring, the practicing in front of the mirror, the repetition of movements and positions, the attention paid to form, the getting up every day and going to the gym and doing it over and over—all of this is part of the creation process of a muscle memory. Even the music blaring in the gym plays a role, for music activates the same areas of the brain as those associated with memory making—a certain song, played over and over, therefore, may help make a certain movement stick. With so many factors in play, I find myself trying to put my finger on the primary one. Is it repetition? Is it mimicking the movements? Is it purely the feeling you have when it is right—almost an emotion—that sets the memory in neurochemical concrete?

Paul says that boxing is like calculus. "It doesn't make sense until something just clicks, and then you understand it." No, wait, I think he put it the other way: "It doesn't make sense until you understand it, and then something just clicks." Yes, that was it; it's like a Zen koan: *It doesn't make sense until you understand it.*

And then: *click.*

Today we spent a full hour shadowboxing and then doing drills and calisthenics. I was near the front and felt in sync with Ken in all his movements. I remember watching his feet during one set and knowing that my feet were going at the exact same rhythm, a rhythm that was also in sync with the music. My body had this stuff memorized—the combinations, the shuffle, the jumping jacks, all sharp and precise.

Thursday, April 17

Five weeks down, one week to go. I have definitely improved—I mean, I can jump rope, I can block some punches, land others, do the drills and combinations, hit the bag, and I can certainly keep up with all the running and calisthenics—I can wrap my hands, for God's sake!—but even so, it's still as hard as it was the first week. As in life, what's hard has simply changed. The stakes are higher—boot camp is almost over, and the pressure's on to get better fast. People aren't holding back. The energy is more intense. Guys are getting bloodied. The punches are harder. That's the main thing: The punches are harder.

I had a scary moment yesterday with a sparring partner that made me seriously question what the hell I am doing. He popped me hard several times, so hard I was dazed. I lost my bearings and he was baiting me—"Come on! Come on, man, bring it on!" I came toward him. He punched me again between the eyes. This time, I fell to the ground. I got back up. Now I was just pissed. I kept my right glove glued to my face—I could feel it there—and when he started jabbing at me, I slipped and rolled under it and kept moving around him in circles. I kept moving until the bell went off, ending the round. He never got another shot at me.

A little rage: Maybe that's what I needed.

I had also taken to heart something Paul said one morning: "It's not *natural*—boxing's not natural." He paced back and forth in front of the mirror. "Your instinct is to thrust your chest *out*"—he did so—"and hold your head *up*!" He looked laughable now, like a peacock, strutting. "But a *boxer*"—still pacing, he shot us a glance, which silenced everyone—"a boxer has to contort his body, keep his chin *down*, head down, elbows in, fists here," at his jaw. "He's *street*, man. He's lookin' for a fight. And if you give him shit"—Paul threw a lightning fast jab—"you'll be sorry."

I didn't think I could quite pull this off—I'd need another six months of boxing boot camp—but I could almost picture it.

Monday, April 21

The final challenge I face as boot camp comes to a close is with my hitting—hitting with all my might. I have the muscle, I have the technique, but I hold back. The coaches see this and grow frustrated: "I want to see a *full* extension, Billy! When you jab, push out that arm *all* the way. Punch it *out*!"

The power of a hit is not in the fist. I know this now. It needs to come from the entire back and rotating trunk—the whole upper body—and shoot out *through* the arm as it unfolds and extends, as one unleashes a punch. That's the secret. And it *does* come when I do it correctly, while shadowboxing or with the bag, when I stretch my arm as far as possible, with a hard, sharp, clean precision—the power, but also something more—a certain grace, an elegance to the line. A boxer's jab, in this way, is like a ballet dancer's extension. But connecting on a punch depends on more than technique. It starts in the head. You have to feel like you can do it, want to do it—need to, have to.

This morning I was in the ring with the skinny, gangly dude with tattoos everywhere. We were both suited up in full protective gear. Tat Man was as tall as the redhead and just as experienced a boxer, if not more, but his eyes weren't cold. Immediately, he started coaching me. "Get in there, come closer, I'll block, you hit—"

I jabbed at his trunk. Tat Man backed away, smiling. "Try it again," he told me, "but harder. You're hardly tapping me."

I shuffled in and threw a few punches—

"Good, good, but harder, keep going."

I did, and I got better. Hitting the trunk was easier psychologically for the simple fact that you're *not* hitting the face, the head—the brain. But now he told me to take a shot with all my might.

"Hit me. Go ahead, just hit me."

I did, right to the forehead.

"No, harder."

Again.

"Okay, but *harder*. To my face. Hard. Hit me in the face as hard as you possibly can, man."

How often in life does one hear someone say that?

"Really?"

He nodded. I felt like I should make sure there were witnesses to it.

Okay, what the hell: I made his right temporal lobe a target and went at it with my glove. I hit him again and again and again, but the funny thing was, it was as if I could not hit him hard enough. I mean that in two ways. I just couldn't hit him 100 percent full force—80 percent maybe but not 100. I still held something back: I didn't want to hurt him, break his nose, knock him out, cause a concussion. At the same time, there was some crazy glint in his eyes. He actually liked getting punched. I could probably never hit hard enough to satisfy him.

The bell rang: time to switch sparring partners.

I paired up with the chunky white guy with the white patches in his brown hair. I wanted to keep the rhythm going I had with Tat Man. I barreled in and threw a bunch of body hits. I was not swinging wildly but landing hits and riding a surge of adrenaline—or perhaps it had nothing to do with neurochemistry at all or, for that matter, with understanding. It was just confidence, confidence alone: knowingness unhitched from intellect or emotion, like when you're on a bike and ride hands-free. No questions, no second thoughts, no remembering, no trying, just doing: this is what I had sought.

It was a rush, not unlike the feeling one sometimes gets while having sex—a feeling of physical power, one body dominating another. What made it better was that my opponent was putting up a fight, trying to fend me off. I could see it in his body. I could see it in his face, red and drenched in sweat beneath the headgear. He was holding his own, but he looked overwhelmed. Or was it surprised? He stepped back and spit out his mouth guard and caught his breath: "You are *pumped*, man."

Yes I am, I thought to myself.

"Okay? You ready?" I said and I charged toward him.

Library Rats

The erudite body is a good body to have.

—COLIN MCGINN, *SPORT*, 2008

After my meeting with Vivian Nutton, I'd left London with a new lead in my mission to investigate Mercuriale's *Gymnastica*. Dr. Nutton's translation of the work was the first in English, but it was not the first, period. An Italian version was done in 1960 on the occasion of the Rome Olympics, and some forty years later, a contemporary French scholar published a critical edition of the *Gymnastica* with a partial translation in French. The scholar, Jean-Michel Agasse, subsequently published a number of academic papers on aspects of Mercuriale's life and work, articles he later revised and contributed—translated from the French—to the volume containing Dr. Nutton's translation. The two had worked together closely on the project, and his name came up several times during our conversation. I picked up that there was a certain difference in their approaches. "Jean-Michel knows more about Mercuriale than I do,"

Dr. Nutton acknowledged, "and really has dedicated his life to him." Pause. "He's a Mercuriale nut."

That clinched it: I knew I had to meet this person.

Dr. Nutton made an introduction, and Jean-Michel Agasse responded to my email with surprising alacrity (perhaps because "Girolamo Mercuriale" was in the subject line). Though he lived in a tiny village in the Pyrenees ("Eighty kilometers from the nearest town, close to Lourdes, the city of the Holy Virgin," he noted), as luck would have it, he would be in Paris for the next several days.

My whole approach to travel at that time was not unlike my approach to street photography: to remain open to chance and trust my instincts. So I bought a ticket to Paris and arranged to stay at a friend's apartment in St. Germain.

The day before our meeting, I received a message from Monsieur Agasse suggesting that we meet at a café near the Luxembourg Gardens. "Now," he added, "as in all good spy stories, how shall we recognize each other? I am (almost) bald, have a moustache and glasses, and shall wear a white jacket. This should be enough."

I told him that I would wear a fedora and dark glasses.

I FOUND MONSIEUR Agasse sitting at an outdoor table and sipping an espresso. As we exchanged pleasantries and began to get acquainted, I instantly noticed that he was French in exactly the same way that Vivian Nutton was English, which is to say, in an almost exaggerated yet unselfconscious way—the gestures, the mannerisms, the appearance, the distinctive accent, even their names. If Dr. Nutton was a real Mr. Chips, Jean-Michel was straight out of a Truffaut film, brooding and poetical and elegantly rumpled in his unstructured white jacket.

He had taught Latin for many years in a high school in the Pyrenees, he told me, but as he got older and more and more tired of dealing with the parents of his students—always more difficult than the children—he decided to get an advanced degree. This was about fifteen years ago; he was in his midsixties now. One day he happened upon Mercuriale in a small book on "Neo-Latin," the more refined form of the Latin in use during the medieval period and largely employed for scholarly publications starting around 1500. This led him to the *Gymnastica*, which became the subject of his doctoral thesis. "I opened the book and thought, 'This is what I'm going to do.' I loved the illustrations," Jean-Michel added with a sheepish look.

"We have that in common," I told him.

"I am a comic strip reader, so I guess that's one reason why." A fan of Art Spiegelman, Chris Ware, and other contemporary graphic novel artists, he was equally enamored of the more traditional American pop culture comics: X-Men, Superman, Batman, Spider-Man. He read and collected them all. And indeed, the godlike athletic figures depicted in the *Gymnastica*, with their bulging muscles, would not have been out of place in a superhero universe.

The artist whom Mercuriale had commissioned to do these drawings, as I'd learned some time earlier, was a complicated character named Pirro Ligorio. The two had known each other for a decade, having met when Mercuriale first joined the Farnese household in Rome, but they were different in many respects. Ligorio, a hotheaded Neapolitan twenty years older than Mercuriale, lacked the physician's innate diplomatic skills—essential for surviving in the elite cultural and curial circles in Rome—and fell out of favor with the papal court. He'd found refuge in the court of the Duke of Ferrara when he heard from his old friend sometime around 1572. To an extent neither man could ever have predicted, Ligorio's dynamic drawings would give the *Gymnastica* a life long beyond their own.

Unlike me, Jean-Michel was immediately able to move beyond Ligorio's images and read Mercuriale's text in the original Latin. He found it resonated with a number of his interests, academic and personal. "Since a very, very long time, the real thing in which I am interested is the body. *What does it mean to have a body?*"

Both of his parents were medical doctors, Jean-Michel told me, so perhaps a certain curiosity had been passed on. But his interest in the body as a young man was not clinical—he could never imagine studying anatomy, dissecting cadavers, as I once had—but instead, philosophical. He practiced yoga and meditation, which he learned when he lived in India and studied with a master. In the seventies, he traveled to the United States and got into primal scream therapy and encounter groups. He tried it all. Part of it was the times, and part of it was his upbringing. "I was raised as a Catholic, and even as a child I had the feeling that the body was really forgotten; it was something put apart. I suppose that all these years I've been in search of my own body."

Studying Mercuriale provided a way to explore this from a historical perspective. During the Middle Ages, the emphasis was on the soul, one's spiritual life. The body—which had been idealized, fetishized, by the Greeks—was now seen more as a vessel for sin. Exercise was considered self-indulgent. But this changed with the rise of humanism in the fourteenth century, Jean-Michel explained: "They get out of the very dark way of seeing in the Catholic church, and see that the body is something beautiful," as the Greeks had. "Taking care of oneself—the sense of the individual—returns." And not necessarily in a purely secular way: "It's linked with one's relationship to God," he said. Mercuriale's passion for exercise made more sense in this context.

Even so, Mercuriale had to be careful, as Jean-Michel made clear. The Council of Trent, convened in 1545 to begin addressing the reforms demanded by Martin Luther, was nearing its conclusion when Mercuriale started work; his book would have to pass muster with church authorities. What's remarkable, really, is that Mercuriale's treatise wasn't more infused with Catholic dogma. Which is not to say that it's secular exactly, but instead that it is intended first and foremost as a medical text. Of the hundreds of sources he references on the topic of exercise, hygiene, and the body, the Bible is not among them.

Given his connection to Cardinal Farnese, Mercuriale would have had little trouble gaining access to the Vatican Library, which even at this early stage in its history (it was founded less than a hundred years before) held one of the richest collections of ancient Greek, Latin, and Hebrew manuscripts in existence. The scholar Onofrio Panvinio, an Augustinian monk who served as the librarian of the Farnese family library, also aided him in his research, procuring texts for him. (The Farnese library was housed within the great Palazzo Farnese, a short walk from the cardinal's official residence, an equally grand palazzo called the Cancelleria, where Mercuriale also lived.) What's more, Mercuriale himself was an avid collector of books, so much so that he would later confess to a colleague that he suffered from "bibliomania."

By the time he retired back in Forli, Mercuriale had a personal library of about twelve hundred books, primarily medical texts, all carefully inventoried. However, they have long since disappeared, Jean-Michel told me. He had spent years trying to track them down without success. "It seems they are nowhere. You would think there would be a mark on the books, a stamp, marking them as his—ex libris, Hieronymous Mercurialis." Jean-Michel suspected that they were destroyed—trashed when Napoleon's troops entered north Italy, for instance, but who knows? "Maybe they still sleep some-where in an unknown library," he said with a hopeful smile. "This is an enigma that is still to be solved."

If he sounded like a bit of a sleuth, well, he was. In his spare time, Jean-Michel liked to write detective stories. He certainly didn't spend it working out. As with Vivian Nutton, working on the *Gymnastica* had no impact on his exercise routine. A little snow skiing, yes, some horseback riding in summer, but that was it—and he wasn't a sports fan. "I like being *le rat de bibliothèque*—how do you say?—'library rat,' something like that. There is something sensual about having old books. For me, my first experience of that was at the Vatican Library—"

"—like Mercuriale," I said.

Jean-Michel nodded. "I remember having these papers from the sixteenth century—the materiality of it was moving for me. To be able to turn the pages and know that it was five hundred years old, that someone had written this with their own hand. It carries this evidence of the body, and of the different bodies involved. It is like carrying their bodies still, the oils from their hands—the sweat."

JEAN-MICHEL AND I left the café and walked together for a few blocks. We parted ways near the Sorbonne, where he ducked into a small bookshop specializing in philosophy and psychoanalysis. I headed for one of my favorite museums, L'Orangerie, where eight of Claude Monet's *Water Lilies* live in two linked circular rooms. The canvases line the entire perimeter; it's like being inside an aquarium of impressionism.

I had come not only to immerse myself in Monet but also to get some moderate exercise of a sort recommended by an Italian doctor who followed in Mercuriale's footsteps, Giulio Mancini. Born in 1559, Mancini was a medical man who moonlighted in art—he was a canny art dealer, most notably of the paintings of Caravaggio. And he advocated visiting "picture galleries" as a way to combine recreation for body, soul, and mind alike. He felt that art galleries were ideal settings for strolling in an enclosed space. This notion wasn't entirely new. Porticoes designed expressly for walking were incorporated into public and private space going back to ancient Greece.

Mancini's English contemporary Robert Burton, in his 1621 door-stopper *The Anatomy of Melancholy*, recommended taking up the study of art (as well as maps, jewels, antiquities, or beautiful objects of any kind) as an antidote to grief. In Burton's words, "Amongst those exercises, or recreations of the mind within doors, there is none so general, so aptly to be applied to all sorts of men, so fit and proper to expel Idleness and Melancholy, as that of Study." And Mercuriale himself wholeheartedly supported walking as an ideal form of exercise—preferably in verdant outdoor settings, where he felt that taking in the sight of flowers and foliage literally sharpened one's eyesight. But Mancini, the personal physician to several cardinals in Rome, combined the prescriptions of both men.

Landscape painting was Mancini's preferred vehicle for this form of exercise—for its transporting and transcendent qualities—a genre that Monet's water lilies don't exactly fall into. But I have no doubt the doctor would have approved. I took two leisurely laps around the circular galleries at L'Orangerie—equivalent to a few blocks, I'd guess—then went down to the larger, longer rectangular galleries (filled with a variety of impressionist artists' work) before returning upstairs. I sat in each room once, twice, and was just about to leave, then went back for a third time, knowing that I probably would not return for many years to L'Orangerie, if at all. This time, I walked as close to the walls as possible and instead of looking at the paintings themselves, I studied the borders, where the canvas meets the frame. I was surprised to see that Monet painted to the very edges and beyond, right onto the gold frame itself, as if filling in every last patch with color. If you look closely, you might think it looks messy. After all, he could have wiped the frame clean. But no, I thought to myself: that is how to paint, as it is how to live—to the very borders. Make a mess of it if you must. Just don't leave anything blank.

I left the museum and began walking through the streets of Paris. I walked for an hour, then two. Dead tired and parched as the sun was setting, I ended up in a bar in the Marais, where, serendipitously, drinks were on the house because of an art exhibit opening there (combining two other forms of recreation, I thought to myself with approval). And the house was packed.

The bartender, who looked astonishingly like a young David Bowie, inquired what I was doing in Paris, and I tried to explain. Something got lost in translation—or the din—for he was convinced that I had said I was writing a book on the history of exorcism.

"Ah, you are good friends with Linda Blair, then?" he noted casually, as he pushed a half-pint in my direction.

A Duel

We are what we repeatedly do.
Excellence, then, is not an act but a habit.

—ARISTOTLE (384–322 B.C.)

C ertain forms of exercise Mercuriale could not recommend
because they had not been dreamed up yet—aerobics, Pilates,
running on a treadmill. About others, such as wrestling and boxing,
he had understandable qualms; the potential for harm could far
outweigh potential benefits to one's health. But there was one activity
he was unable to recommend or even write about at length because,
in its most extreme form, it had been condemned by the Council of
Trent: the art of fencing.

Training and fighting with swords developed in the Western
world during the Bronze Age, the period beginning roughly around
3200 B.C., which also saw the rise of city-states and the first writing
systems. One can see examples of such crude ancient weapons at
museums, but to my mind they remain objects, collecting dust, life-
less, bloodless, in such settings. They are made more real somehow

in the dynamic fictional world of Homer, where swords, spears, axes, and shields figure almost like minor characters. This is especially so in the *Iliad*, the written version of which dates to the mid-eighth century B.C., but is set some five centuries earlier during the Trojan War. Early on in the story, Paris—the handsome lug who triggered the entire death-littered epic by seducing Helen, the wife of Menelaus, king of Sparta—challenges "the best and the bravest" of the Greeks to a duel. Helen, characterized as the ultimate trophy wife, will be the victor's prize, thereby also bringing an end to the war. Who should step forward to accept the challenge—actually, he leaps from his chariot—but the cuckold in question: Lord Menelaus. Paris blanches and recoils into the crowd. But it's too late to back down now.

As both armies stand back to watch, "Paris quickly put on his resplendent armor. First, he strapped the bronze greaves to his lower legs and fastened them onto his ankles with silver clasps. Next, on his chest he put the finely wrought breastplate of his brother Lycaon, which fitted his body too. Over his shoulder he slung his silver-bossed sword and above it his massive shield. And last he put on his bronze helmet with its blood-chilling horsehair crest, then chose a powerful spear that fitted his hand. In just the same way, Menelaus prepared for battle."

Paris, who'd won the toss-up for first strike, takes his best shot. Menelaus deflects, hurls his spear—a near miss—then charges forward and brings his "great silver-bossed sword" down on Paris's bronze helmet. Victory is virtually his. But, not so fast; the gods have other plans: Zeus allows the sword to shatter and Aphrodite sweeps in, whisks Paris off, and puts him to bed with Helen. This battle is just heating up.

Following the *Iliad*, one of the earliest works to deal with actual, as opposed to mythological, sword fighting is the Roman historian Vegetius's *De re militari* (*On the Military*, also known as *Epitoma rei militaris*), a four-volume opus on Roman military training and strategy. The manuscript dates to the late fourth century A.D., but the first printed editions came over a thousand years later. Vegetius (full name: Publius Flavius Vegetius Renatus) was a kind of Mercuriale of military training who drew primarily on antiquarian sources, but he also describes what seem to be actual military exercises of his day and age, in which he participated. He writes of practicing sword work against a post and fencing with other soldiers as preparation for battle. The Romans, he writes, preferred the thrust over the cut because cuts can be stopped by armor and bone, whereas puncture wounds kill by piercing vital organs directly. This strategy would later be central to Italian and French schools of fencing during the Renaissance.

Knowledge of fencing, as necessary off the battlefield as on, for noblemen as much as for knights, would become a criterion of the ideal gentleman in the vision of the Italian writer Baldesar Castiglione. In his influential 1528 work *The Book of the Courtier*, he writes: "I wish our courtier to be well built, with finely proportioned members, and I would have him demonstrate strength and lightness and suppleness and be good at all the physical exercises befitting a warrior. Here, I believe, his first duty is to know how to handle expertly every kind of weapon . . . and to be especially well informed about all those weapons commonly used among gentlemen. For apart from their use in war, when perhaps the finer points may be neglected, often differences arise between one gentleman and another and lead to duels, and very often the weapons used are those that come immediately to hand. So, for safety's sake, it is important to know about them."

It all sounds gentlemanly, an abstraction somehow. But lest one forget, the intent in a duel was not just to win but to kill. Dueling over questions of honor increased so greatly by the late fifteenth century that the Council of Trent moved to enact severe penalties against it. It decreed that "the detestable custom of dueling which the Devil had originated, in order to bring about at the same time the ruin of the soul and the violent death of the body, shall be entirely uprooted from Christian soil." According to the council, those who took part in a duel were automatically excommunicated, and if killed, denied a Christian burial.

In the aftermath of these rulings, fencing evolved into an art, a martial art, and over the centuries made the transition from military practice to an esoteric athletic event that would be part of the modern Olympic Games—not to mention, competitive high school and college sports programs. Fencing is considered a full-body exercise, with special emphasis placed on the musculature of the arms and legs. But it's the deliberative mental agility required to score a "touch" that sets it apart from other combat-based activities like boxing, wrestling, or judo. "Physical chess," it's been called, aptly highlighting that fencing is as much an intellectual as a physical workout.

Back in the sixteenth and seventeenth centuries, fighting with swords became a popular form of entertainment in northern European countries—granted, for men alone—something associated more with an aesthete than a warrior. In this phase, the art of fencing intersected with the history of the printed book. One of the most extravagant and lavishly illustrated volumes produced was an eccentric manual on swordsmanship published in 1630. Known as *Academie de l'Espée*, it was written in French by a fencing master with a name so fancy it sounds straight out of *The Three Musketeers*: Gérard Thibault d'Anvers. (His elaborate appellation, as well as the book's language of origin, has led to the misapprehension that he was French, but in fact he was Dutch. *Anvers* is the French word for Antwerp.) He died before his masterpiece—an endless production— could be finished. Legendary now, the book was so extravagant and expensive—and also, significantly, so large in its dimensions—that only a small number were published, and copies are hard to come by today. I learned that one exists in a public library in Paris, and the day after I met with Jean-Michel Agasse I set out to find it. My destination: the Bibliothèque Nationale de France.

TO CALL IT a library doesn't seem quite right. Libraries, plural, would be more accurate: two enormous modernist high-rises separated by a vast plaza, one that would be perfect, it struck me, for a duel. The buildings looked identical, and there were no obvious signs indicating a difference between the two. I didn't know where to go at first, so I just picked one and headed in. The entrance was at the bottom of a long, languorous moving sidewalk sloping down. I passed through security and found my way to the history section on the third floor. A security guard sat before a closed door. She told me something very emphatically in French. It seemed highly important—that I grasped right away—but it was several minutes and a game of charades before I figured out that she was saying I needed to have a library card to gain access. Perfectly reasonable, but I was in the wrong building: "Est," she said, five or six times, louder each time, as if I could not hear her. "Est, est, est, est!"

"Est, yes, *east*, I understand." I made my way out of that high-rise, back up the moving sidewalk, across the enormous plaza and into the other building.

I went through security and headed to the information desk. I showed the woman seated there the paper I'd printed out from the library's online catalog with details on the fencing book. She studied it, and gave me a sour and skeptical look. "Why?" she said. That's all she said. She started typing on her computer, as if she had far more important things to do than listen to my answer.

I told her I'm conducting research on exercise. I told her something about the book in question. She ceased typing. Again, a skeptical look. It wasn't that she didn't understand English, she clearly did; it was more like she didn't know what I was talking about—or care. *Exercise? Fencing?* Regardless, she instructed me to go to the Research Office, near the bookshop. She pointed in a vaguely eastern direction. I thanked her and turned.

"I wish you a good luck," she said grimly.

I didn't spot an office near the bookshop, so I kept looking. I walked and walked and walked down an empty corridor, at least half a block long, thinking it must be coming up at any moment yet also feeling it was too late to go back to where I'd started. I turned corners and kept walking. I started to feel unaccountably exhausted. Soon, Aristotle—or rather, a book credited to Aristotle—sprang to mind.

"Why are long walks on level ground more fatiguing than over uneven ground, but short ones are less fatiguing?" he asked in his book *Problems*. "Is it because prolonged and vigorous movement produces fatigue? [And] why does the road seem to be longer, when we walk without knowing how long it is, than when we know . . . ? Is it because to know how long it is, is to know its number, and the infinite is always greater than the determinate?"

As it turned out, I had a tremendous amount of time to consider this problem for myself. The corridors seemed endless. To turn around would have been pointless, so I distracted myself from the vaguely existential meaninglessness of what I was doing by considering the act of walking itself. "If there is one kind of exercise which is most of all to be sought and practiced by those who are concerned about their health," Mercuriale declared, "then it is beyond all doubt that it must be walking." And yet, he noted, "there are only a few who really understand" how it works.

One might consider walking the simplest of exercises. But this is hardly so, as someone who has to regain the ability to walk would certainly know. Some two dozen major muscles of the lower body are involved in every cycle of walking—a cycle being the split-second from the contact of one foot on the ground to the next contact of the

same foot. And far more is happening than simply forward locomo-
tion. A physical therapist once put it to me this way: "Think of
walking as a series of aborted falls." The muscles of the hips, legs,
and feet are just as involved in keeping one from collapsing as they
are in keeping one moving. The hamstrings—the long powerful
muscles on the back of the legs—are chiefly responsible here. They
reach their peak of activity as they "arrest movement" at the hip joint
at the moment the heel strikes the ground. The quadriceps femoris—
the bundle of four muscles otherwise known as the thigh—then
begin to contract to control the load being imposed on the knee joint
by the body.

After about twenty-five minutes, I found myself heading toward
the information desk and the woman who'd wished me "a good luck."
I'd walked around the entire complex without realizing it. Silly as it
sounds, I couldn't face her, having failed to follow her directions.
I tried to slip by her, but librarians know this particular move all too
well; very little escapes their notice. When I looked up, she was
eyeing me over her computer monitor. We locked eyes, and in my
head I could hear her saying in her grim voice: "Why? Why? *Why?*"

I put my head down and kept walking until I spotted a friendly
looking security guard. I showed him my piece of paper and explained
my dilemma. He left his post and walked me to the Research Office,
which was, indeed, near the bookshop—if your definition of "near"
is "behind." There were no signs. In French, he explained what I
needed to the woman behind the desk. I thanked him, he sailed
away, and I took a seat before a gray-haired, elderly woman wearing
a simple gray-patterned dress. I smiled. "Parlez-vous anglais?"

She looked at me with something like pity and said nothing. She
took my paper and studied it carefully, then unleashed a torrent of
French. In my memory, she was actually leaning over the desk, her
face close to mine. She wasn't—she couldn't have been—but that's
how it felt, the force of her words.

I stared back, stricken, guilty: "Désolé, désolé très!" I would have apologized to the entire nation of France for not speaking their language, if I could have. She held up a form, like a prop, and again delivered a speech in French. I took the paper. I couldn't read it, but I guessed that it was asking for my name, address, and so on. I returned it to her, completed. Again, a blank stare. Finally, a single word in English: "Why?"

Why, indeed? I was beginning to wonder myself. I'd never had much interest in fencing myself. It's the use of weaponry—knives, basically—that puts me off. For the same reason, I am not drawn to shooting or archery. If I had to fight, I'd rather do it with my own body. But tracking down this rare volume had become an irresistible challenge, one I had to see through to the end.

"I'm a writer," I replied. "Research. A book. The history of exercise." I smiled helpfully.

Just like her colleague at the information desk, she answered with nothing but a puzzled expression.

"*Sports?*" I added, trying to find some common ground here.

She waved her hand with impatience and began typing. For the first time, I relaxed a bit. I sat back in the chair and looked around. Forgetting that she didn't understand English, I said, thinking out loud, "This library is so remarkable, so remarkable—incredible!"

The gray woman in gray stopped what she was doing and glanced up. She looked squarely at me, and her face softened just a little bit. "Ah, but you have the New York library," she replied in perfect English.

I was taken aback. "Yes, we do! In fact . . ." I reached for my bag and pulled from it my NYPL baseball cap and pushed it on my head. She looked at the hat and at my crazy smile, and she laughed and nodded. "Alors!" She motioned for me to look into the little camera stationed to the upper right. She took my photo—big smile on my face—and moments later handed me my library card. She provided careful instructions about my next steps—paying a fee, coat check, and so forth. I thanked her kindly and proceeded to follow the instructions, and reported back to the Information Woman. She appraised me with a look that said, "You again?"

I did not say a word. I simply placed the red BNF library card on the desk before her. Victory. She picked it up and studied it carefully, looking at the photo, then me, the photo, then me. I just waited, smiling the same crazy smile as in my photograph. "Alors," she finally declared. She took out a map of the library and began charting my course. I got a second wind. I listened carefully to everything the Information Woman said and followed her finger as she traced the somewhat complicated route I was still to take. At last, she finished. "I wish you a good luck," she murmured, as grimly as before.

From there, I walked through a turnstile, down an escalator as long as those in the London Underground, and through another hallway until I came to a room grander than any I had yet encountered, identified by a large sign with nothing but the letter *T* (*as in Temple?*). I tiptoed up to the dais where four librarians were stationed, all looking deeply preoccupied, like priests involved in preparing a ritual of some sort. I surveyed them quickly. One wore a white shirt unbuttoned a little too far, revealing a gold medallion, and had gel in his hair: definitely gay. I went straight to him and showed him my paper with the listing for the fencing book. "Ah, yes, darling, right this way," he said soothingly. He came around the desk and guided me to a set of steel doors, emblazoned with the words "La Reserve des livres rares."

"Right through here, then take the lift to L-3," he said, then repeated it. "L-3, L-trois. Trois."

"Oui, trois," I repeated, and showed him three fingers to confirm I had it right. "Merci, merci beaucoup." Before pushing through door one, I paused, suddenly overwhelmed and confused. I looked at him and said, in all sincerity, "What if I get lost? What if I never find my way back out?"

He looked nonplussed. "We shall come find you."

This didn't register at first.

"*Voila!*" He motioned, as if to say, "Come on, hurry along, time's a-wasting!"

I pushed through the first door, pulled the second, and then took the elevator to L-3. "L-trois," I murmured under my breath. "L-trois, L-trois, L-trois . . ."

The doors opened onto an empty vestibule with one door. It was locked. Within a moment, a click, and it opened automatically onto a reading room as plush as it was silent. I took a deep breath. I was almost there. I could feel it. Merely accessing this one treasured book and navigating this vast library had taken me almost my entire day yet also honed sparring skills I didn't even know I possessed. I pulled out my piece of paper, now crumpled, and presented it to one of the librarians. He read it carefully and gave me a form to fill out. When I handed it back, he replied, "You are number twenty-two." He gave me a key and told me to put the few things I had with me—pad, pencil, laptop—into a locker underneath the desk. "You have half an hour," he whispered. By now, it was five o'clock, and this room would be closing at five thirty.

I sat at place number twenty-two, at a highly polished table that looked as though it were made out of a redwood tree. Five other readers sat around the beautiful table, all studying ancient books propped onto red velvet bookstands. It was like being in a luxe monastery; Onofrio Panvinio would have been right at home here, reading illuminated manuscripts. Not two minutes passed before, suddenly, there was a kind of rustle—something breaking the silence, as if a bird flapped its wings or a deer darted by. Out of the corner of my right eye, I saw a figure approaching me: a very large man, perhaps six-foot-five, with long brown hair and a bushy beard. He had not been with the other librarians at the front desk. He wore simple dark clothes. He could have stepped straight out of the Middle Ages, a knight without his suit of armor. He was carrying a book of about three by three and a half feet.

I wondered if this was his sole occupation: Only very large men were qualified to carry such large books.

He came straight toward me with a penetrating gaze, as if he recognized me, and placed the book atop one of the red velvet book-stands with great delicacy. His hands were the size of his face. He opened the tome to the middle page, stepped back, and made a small gesture, like a bow. He never said a word. I whispered a "merci," and he retreated backward. Remarkable! After all this time and waiting and dead ends, the book I had hoped to see arrived within one hundred seconds. I looked over at the librarians behind the desk, wondering if they would give me a conspiratorial smile, as if to say, "Congratulations, you made it, we were just testing you." But they were all absorbed in their work. Maybe the book had been ordered for me hours before, when I'd first entered the library. I would never know.

I took a moment just to let the whole experience soak in. I felt a certain victory that I had actually found the book, achieved my goal, but that feeling—self-congratulatory—passed quickly to one of privilege. How fortunate I was to be here, in this city, in this library, in this room, at this table, with the opportunity to look at this extraordinary, four-hundred-year-old book. I drank it all in. And then I sniffed. I leaned over to smell the book. Nothing: a sign that it was well taken care of—no odor of mold or mildew. All this security, all these precautions, which seemed like obstacles in my way: They were all worth it, if only to preserve such rare volumes.

I was nervous; my hands were sweating. I dried them on my jeans and pulled on a pair of the white cotton gloves supplied on the table, and I began paging through the book. I had only twenty-five minutes now, and I spent it carefully, letting my eyes search out every corner of every one of the thirty-three spreads. The book was a detailed "how-to" on fighting specifically with the rapier—a long, thin, sharp, two-edged sword popular in the sixteenth and seventeenth centuries—and illustrated with sumptuous engravings. In each spread, the fencing figures were dressed in garb from different time periods—ancient Greece, Rome, the Middle Ages, the Renaissance—making it look more like a fanciful history of costume through the ages.

But make no mistake: This was about highly serious swordplay. Death was the point, not beauty. The only thing missing was the impaled bodies. Spread after spread, the figures appeared to be going through an entire duel, meticulously mapped, as if a movie of a dance performance were broken down into each of its individual frames. The author had employed an elaborate theory in which geometry was applied to fencing footwork using an imaginary circle—"The Mysterious Circle," he called it—that made little immediate sense to me. But the bookmaking artistry involved was undeniable. What a shame that Gérard Thibault d'Anvers did not live to see his *Academie de l'Espèe* in print.

At five thirty I carefully closed the book, stepped back from the table, notified the librarian that I'd finished, retrieved my belongings, and retraced my steps. I made two brief stops before exiting. I waved to the gay librarian in the T section and blew him a kiss, and I stopped at the information desk on my way out. "I wish you a good luck," I said genuinely to the woman seated behind the counter. She nodded and returned silently to her work.

Outside, it was pouring rain. I used my umbrella as a rapier and gave it a modest lunge, then walked slowly across the long plaza to the Metro.

On the Nature of Running

Eating alone will not keep a man well; he must also take exercise . . .
Those who get exhausted with running should wrestle,
And those who get exhausted with wrestling should run.

—HIPPOCRATES, CA. 400 B.C.

Back in New York, what comes to mind as I go for a run is one of my favorite lines from Mercuriale: "Running is supreme."
Of course it is.

I make this my mantra:

Running is supreme, I think, as I wait for a light to change green in front of my building.

Running is supreme: as I dodge cars and dogs on leashes and bicyclists on the sidewalk.

Running is supreme: as I reach the Hudson and head down the West Side of Manhattan on a smoothly paved path.

What made running supreme in Mercuriale's mind was not only that it met the definition for exercise he carefully laid out in his book, but that it is "granted to all." Anyone is capable of doing it—man, woman, child. One doesn't need a gymnasium. One doesn't need equipment or an opponent. (Not even shoes are necessary, some today say, following the longtime practice of the Tarahumara Indians of Mexico, although ultimately one's feet may disagree.) One needs only healthy lungs and a pair of reasonably strong legs. I am acutely conscious of mine as they run, how they do this automatically. But I also find myself enjoying willing them to do what I like, as if I were driving a car. I take a right and run to the end of a pier. I run backward, then forward, and then steer back to where I began. I never look down. Each of my feet will touch the ground a thousand times, at least, perhaps twice that, for every mile I cover, while absorbing three times my body weight. I pick up my pace. I spot someone running more slowly than me and deliberately overtake him. It feels good to feel fast. This is my own private version of endurance running, which, some evolutionary biologists argue, may explain how we came to run in the first place.

It wasn't a given that being able to stand upright and walk—as early hominids first did some four million or more years ago—would lead to this: this remarkable ability to cover distances great and short at varying speed by one's legs alone. After all, other animals are bipedal—some reptiles, birds, many mammals—but with the exception of a rare few, such as the ostrich, they aren't able to run as humans can. Our close relatives, nonhuman primates—chimpanzees, gibbons, baboons—can move on two feet alone for limited distances (if wounded, say, or if carrying something with the front limbs), but not at marathon lengths, and not at impressive speed. What accounts for this special ability in humans?

Multiple theories have been proposed to explain our leap to two feet. (*Leap* being a relative term: We are talking about changes that took place over millennia.) Some biologists argue that it was the transition from living in dense jungle to open savanna habitats that gave those who could stand upright a distinct survival advantage.

They could now navigate visually, reach higher when foraging, carry food while walking, and move more rapidly—less vulnerably—over the plains. Others see in bipedalism a defense strategy—the ability to stand and make oneself seen and heard to ward off predators. Distinct advantages for the female may have come into play, too—an upright posture making the weight of pregnancy easier for the lower spine to bear, for example. These and other theories are not mutually exclusive; a number of selective forces may have collectively driven the development of bipedalism. But, conceivably, it could have ended there. If early humans could have survived by walking alone, they would have. Nature takes a wait-and-see attitude. Extra energy is expended as a last resort. The ability to run evolved out of life-or-death necessity, no doubt, not as an added bonus for those who are finished foraging for the day and bored with walking. And it was most likely spurred by a dramatic shift in eating habits.

With gradual changes to the climate and their environment, early humans had to supplement a vegetarian diet with a carnivorous one. And in the absence of efficient weapons for a quick kill, they had to become adept at what is now called persistence hunting. This means exactly what it sounds like: chasing after animals and running them into exhaustion and/or heatstroke, at which point they finally wind up as dinner. This could take days. To outrun wild game, early humans had to have an edge over animals in numerous anatomical ways. And eventually we did, starting right at the top, with a head that remains stable while running, not flopping around. Additionally, we developed the ability to breathe efficiently while moving at a fast clip; large gluteus muscles to keep the trunk steady; short toes to aid in balancing; longer limbs; agile ankles; and an Achilles tendon to put a spring in our step. But there is also this, something perhaps less obvious as an evolutionary adaptation and, I daresay, less appreciated: sweat.

Many of us may view sweating as a nuisance or embarrassment, something to be stopped, sopped up, apologized for, covered over with deodorants, ended with Botox. I often get the impression, too, that some people don't understand its primary purpose. One hears men and women alike say they want to "sweat out the toxins" (or the alcohol drunk the night before) in a sauna, or that they exercise expressly to work up a good sweat and "cleanse the system," detox by way of aerobics or hot yoga. But this is a misconception. We have other organs in our body that serve that purpose—namely, the liver and kidneys. Filtering out toxins and wastes is their primary job. While a minuscule amount of cellular waste is secreted in sweat, this is incidental. The primary function of sweat glands is thermo-regulation. We sweat mainly because our core temperature has risen. The fluid secreted onto the skin through pores provides a medium for evaporative cooling: an ingenious—and remarkably effective—form of instant air conditioning. Those who insist that there must be other health benefits to sweating, such as flushing out toxins, are missing the point. The benefit of sweating is that it keeps you from dying.

Current research suggests that there is not a direct relationship per se between being bipedal and the development of sweat glands. Instead, sweating likely evolved to aid survival in hot desert climates. For this, early ancestors such as Lucy, the so-named fossilized remains of a walking hominid, eventually had to lose their furry coats. Don't get me wrong. There are many advantages to being hairy (and I speak from experience): Thick fur provides a barrier against sun, rain, and cold, and protects from thorns and brush. But in the long run—and I mean that in both senses of the phrase—less hair proved to be more advantageous for primitive hunter-gatherers on the move. Gradually, thick body hair was lost, except where it was beneficial as a secondary sexual characteristic—hair on the scalp and pubis being the human equivalent to brightly colored feathers on a bird. Naked skin turned out to be ideal, but there was an evolu-tionary catch: It had to be kept cool.

Two main types of sweat glands evolved: apocrine and eccrine (both words derive from a Greek root for *secretion*). The apocrine gland is embedded deep in the skin, always adjacent to a hair follicle, and produces a viscous fluid that coats the hair shaft. Apocrine glands are concentrated in thickly hairy areas such as the armpit. Bacteria, not the apocrine fluid itself, cause the funky but sometimes-sexy smell that can emanate from here. Eccrine glands are far smaller in size and far more numerous—one has four to six million of these, each opening to the skin's surface through an individual pore. Eccrine glands are our primary agents for cooling; they produce a watery, slightly salty fluid, and are found on every surface of the body except in three extra-sensitive spots: the lips, the ear canal, and the outermost portions of sexual organs—the head of the penis and the clitoris. They are most prevalent on the palms, soles of the feet, and forehead.

Anatomically, the eccrine sweat gland is simplicity itself—just a tube, like the stem of a tiny hydroponic flower turned upside down—but the mechanisms involved to trigger sweating are complex. The equivalent of heat sensors within the skin play a critical moni-toring role, but even so, sweating is more of a neurological function than a dermatological one; it is chiefly the brain region called the hypothalamus that controls regulation of body temperature.

Sweat glands are formed in utero, all several million of them. They are fully intact at birth, so sweating can be detected within the first few days of life—if not the first hours. What one may see and feel an infant experience right away is what is called emotional sweating—sweating triggered by pain, fear, anger, panic, nervous-ness, any powerful emotion. Even ecstasy, I suppose. While thermal sweating occurs over the entire body, emotional sweating is confined to the forehead, armpits, soles of the feet, and palms. The same glands used for cooling are involved, but under different circum-stances. Like thermal sweating, emotional sweating evolved in early hominids most likely as part of the fight-or-flight response. Having damp palms and soles actually aids in gripping if one is on the run, climbing, or throwing—something that athletes know intuitively. This is why baseball players spit in their hands before batting or pitching. As for a dripping-wet forehead, one theory suggests this is a kind of corporeal SOS: a sign, right at eye level and immediately recognizable to others of your kind, that you are in distress—a silent scream spoken in beads of sweat. Wet, odoriferous armpits likely evolved to serve a similar function, communicating emotional states via both the visual and the olfactory systems. At such moments, fear—and desire—really can be smelled.

Emotional sweating is found in humans and animals alike, as Charles Darwin observed: "When a man suffers from an agony of pain, the perspiration often trickles down his face; and I have been assured by a veterinary surgeon that he has frequently seen drops falling from the belly and running down the inside of the thighs of horses, and from the bodies of cattle, when thus suffering." A similar response had been observed in a female hippopotamus, whose whole body was "covered with red-colored perspiration while giving birth to her young," Darwin writes. "So it is with extreme fear; the same veterinary has often seen horses sweating from this cause . . . and with man it is a well-known symptom." Indeed, if you were running for your life—a situation presumably not uncommon among our primitive ancestors (when preyed on, say, or fleeing natural disaster or an enemy)—both systems of perspiration, thermal and emotional, would kick in, rendering your flesh as slick and wet as a just-born baby hippopotamus's.

The fossil record reveals much about our evolution as bipeds—but only so much. While bits of bone tell us that early hominids could run and did run (undoubtedly because they had to run), what's left unsaid is whether they sometimes *chose* to run. Did Lucy and her kind ever run for exercise or pleasure, to use the modern terms?

One can only speculate. Those who deplore running would likely say there's no way that a prehistoric man, woman, or child would go running for no reason other than for the sake of running. But I beg to differ. What I find when I go for a run is that I am conscious of the world, the natural world, in totally different ways than when I am walking. It is uniquely pleasurable. I am conscious of wind, of running against the wind—its force—and of the wind behind me, and of the sun, of its perfectly circular shape, and its heat, its warmness on my body, and the shadow it casts in front of me. I am aware of the ground, the earth, beneath me, and of how changes in terrain register instantly at the soles of my feet. I notice my arms pumping— an action they do not normally do—and the sweat I am generating. But not only my sweat, other fluids as well—nose running, blood coursing, eyes tearing, spit gathering at the corners of my mouth—the inner and outer lubricants of a well-tuned vehicle, as I prefer to see them.

When one is running, time passes differently. I can get from here to there quickly—quickness is embodied, experienced—and I can keep going. I will run until I feel tired, until I've had enough, and then I will go just a little farther, at which point a wave of well-being-ness washes over me. This is not coincidental. My brain is rewarding me for doing something grueling that is beneficial to my overall health—and providing an incentive to do it again. Sustained activity triggers the release of specific neurochemicals, endorphins, which have a kind of tranquilizing effect. On top of that, the body gets a deposit of human growth factor, a repairer of muscle tissue, as well as specialized proteins that, according to new research, are involved in the creation of neurons and the connections between them, synapses. It may even be that being athletic—running, climbing, building muscle—was critical to the increase of mental capacity and brain size in early humans: physical activity as a driver of human intelligence, not the other way around. In other words, I might not be sitting here right now thinking and writing about the nature of running had our earliest ancestors not chosen to go for a run.

EXACTLY WHEN RUNNING became something more than, or other than, a survival strategy is impossible to say with certainty. Some of the earliest recorded instances of running are found in Egyptian wall reliefs dating as far back as 1500 B.C., long before the first Olympic Games were held. A "ritual run" was the central event in a "Jubilee Celebration" during which the reigning pharaoh, whether male or female, strove to regenerate their divine powers through a series of activities and, in so doing, ward off younger, stronger would-be successors to the throne. The ritual run was not of any great distance—it served a symbolic function. But apparently it was demarcated with a "start" and a "finish" line, which brings it into the realm of athletics, albeit with one important exception: there was no competitor, no rival. The pharaoh ran alone, the point being to impress the gods who might magically revitalize them. But the trappings for sports were falling into place. Once established, this ritual run recurred every three years—at Saqqara, a running track was made for this purpose—which suggests a foreshadowing of the competitive athletics that would become an important part of Egyptian and, even more so, Greek culture.

Egyptian runners were invariably depicted in wall reliefs and hieroglyphs wearing the equivalent of shorts or a loincloth. Not so the Greeks, as is well documented. That male athletes competed in the nude is something we accept today without question, more as historical fact than as anomalous behavior. On Greek vases and amphorae we see the images of naked men running, wrestling, and boxing, and engaged in brutal pankration matches (wrestling, boxing, and kicking combined), their genitals exposed. In these depictions, it's as if these tender parts of the body were not tender in the least but tough enough to be knocked around, crushed, jostled, boxed, hit. Or that whatever damage was done was worth it for the sake of the physical performance—to be naked was to be ungirded, unbridled, allowing one to lift more, punch more powerfully, run faster—or, equally, for the sheer beauty of it.

But all of this raises a question: Could this *really* have been so? Could this *be* so? Can one actually run a race without athletic support? How does that work exactly? I had to find out for myself.

My partner, Oliver, had a home in the country on a large piece of land. The nearest neighbors were half a mile away. The driveway alone was a quarter of a mile long—perfect for putting my question to the test. One day, I waited until Oliver took a nap. I did not want an audience beyond birds and trees. I ran first to the end of the driveway and back clothed in running shorts, underwear, T-shirt, socks. This was my control for comparison in my experiment: *perfectly normal*. Then I shucked the shorts, underwear, and shirt. I kept my shoes on, the supposed advantages of barefoot running notwithstanding, and I took off.

There was some jostling down below, some up-and-downing, some definite—what's the right word?—*bouncing*. Yes, bouncing. But within seconds, my testicles retracted and scrotum followed, as if shrink-wrapping my balls, the two now vacuum-packed within the lower abdomen. My penis contracted to a fraction of its normal size. It was as if a message had been sent to the nervous system by wire: *Pack it up quickly, boys.* I found myself sporting nature's own jockstrap.

I ran to the end of the drive and turned around. The sun warmed my whole body and into my insides. I ran my hands over my skin and slopped up the sweat: a manual strigil.

Jogging had passed the test, but what about sprinting? I did roughly a one-hundred-yard dash back to the top of the drive, unbothered by the slight flopping. If anything, I found it comical, how my genitals now resembled a bell, a very small bell, not the least like the church bells Vivian Nutton rang. Beyond this, what I felt deeply was something vital, wild, powerful—more *hunted* than *hunter*: I felt, in a word, like an animal. I turned and sprinted back down the drive as fast as I could.

Mercuriale in Kansas

MITCH: *I am ashamed of the way I perspire. My shirt is sticking to me.*

BLANCHE: *Perspiration is healthy. If people didn't perspire, they would die in five minutes.*

—TENNESSEE WILLIAMS, *A STREETCAR NAMED DESIRE,* 1947

Sometimes I wonder, what would amaze Mercuriale most? That his work is still studied by people like me more than four hundred years after his death? Or, on the contrary: That his work, though appreciated by a small number of scholars, is otherwise completely forgotten and, like him, unknown? He did not become the Galen of his day; instead, he more closely resembles Enoch Soames, the forgotten character trapped in a future he does not recognize in the Max Beerbohm story of the same name.

Would he be amazed that the language in which he wrote, the language he so loved, is now virtually dead, leaving most of his writings inaccessible, unreadable, to most? Or would he be delighted that, even so, an elderly woman in a place called Kansas City, Kansas, in a country called the United States, took it upon herself to translate several of his works into English, and that they were typed up on a little portable machine—a typewriter—itself a form of technology that is already woefully outdated in the digital age? Would he be appalled that the manuscripts haven't seen the light of day in nearly forty years, or would he be pleased that they ended up safely in an archive, which I had come here to see? Surely, Mercuriale would be incredulous that one can fly from New York to Kansas and back within forty-eight hours. (*That one can fly*: It really is amazing, when you stop and think about it for a moment.)

That I was here in Kansas at all was thanks to Arlene Shaner, the Academy of Medicine librarian. When I paid a visit to do research one day, she explained that the Rare Books room was being renovated and ushered me into another room in the library, one I'd never been in before. It was a charmless, large rectangular room with a single long table, like a dining table in an abandoned banquet hall. I took a seat while Ms. Shaner retrieved the books I had put on reserve. One other patron sat on the other side of the table in the otherwise empty room. He wore a terribly serious expression—worry lines creasing his brow—the kind I love to see: the look of someone engaged in something deeply interesting.

Restless, I scanned the shelves behind me. Browsing is a little like fishing, isn't it: Suddenly, my eyes alighted on a gold-embossed title on the spine of a dull-blue book, *Sixteenth Century Physician*, just those three words, and I was hooked. "Physician *singular*," I remember thinking, "*that's odd*." I reached for it and felt a shock of recognition on seeing its full title on the cover: *Sixteenth Century Physician and His Methods: Mercurialis on Diseases of the Skin.*

Mercurialis? My Mercuriale?

Published by a small independent press in Kansas City, Missouri, in 1986, this book had escaped my notice until now. The author, the late Richard L. Sutton, MD, was a dermatologist and professor of dermatology in Kansas City. As he explained in his introduction, he became fascinated by Mercuriale in the mid-1960s and took it upon himself to translate Mercuriale's 1572 book on diseases of the skin, *De morbis cutaneis*, one of the first medical texts on dermatology, with the aim of providing historical context on the Italian doctor's findings. Knowing no Latin did not deter him. He enlisted the help of an Episcopal priest well versed in Latin and a retired school-teacher who had taught Latin in public schools for her entire career, "Miss Irene Blasé," who at age ninety had died one year before his book was published. Sutton went on to explain that Mercuriale's treatise, as originally published, contained two separate works, one on diseases of the skin and one on "excrements"—*De excrementis*, it was titled—but his book dealt solely with the former.

I had known about this other book, but only vaguely. Not knowing Latin and not giving it much thought, I had been under the misim-pression that Mercuriale's treatise on excrements had to do with, well, *excrement*—feces and the bowels—not a subject germane to exercise history. But no: Mercuriale's book on the excrements, Sutton noted, had to do with any substances *excreted* from the human body—feces, urine, sputum, mucus, tears, and sweat. Yes, *sweat*. Given the prevailing belief in humoral theory at the time, this all made perfect sense.

My mind started racing: How could I find an English version of *De excrementis*? What did Mercuriale have to say about sweat? I returned to Sutton's introduction and found him saying, as if speaking directly to me, that Miss Blasé, a "petite maiden lady" with "one good eye," had also done a complete "rough" translation of *De excrementis*, which he intended to deposit in the archives of the Clendening History of Medicine Library, at the University of Kansas Medical Center. Her translation had never been published.

By now, Ms. Shaner had returned with the books I had requested earlier.

I took up the Sutton book and walked to the other end of the room.

"May I interrupt you for a moment?" I whispered to her.

"Of course."

Sometimes I have a hard time explaining things in logical order—I start at the end of a story and go backward, as I did in this instance. Ms. Shaner looked thoroughly confused by whatever I was trying to ask her. I pointed out the passage in Sutton's book and simply let her read it herself. Finally, she smiled and said, "Ah, Dawn McInnis—she's the head archivist at Kansas—the Clendening: wonderful library."

"You know her?"

She looked amused. "It's a small world, the world of rare books librarians. I'll contact her." Ms. Shaner looked at me calmly, as if to say, "Don't get your hopes up. We'll see."

She began typing an email, and I returned to my desk.

I stayed at the library another ninety minutes but found it hard to concentrate. I finally left at about four thirty by which point Ms. Shaner was off "in the stacks," as her colleague told me. I didn't have a chance to say goodbye. When I got home, I received an email bearing good news from Ms. Shaner. The subject line read: *Sweat from De excrementis.*

MY TIMING WAS providential. Dr. Sutton had donated all his papers to the library in 1988, two years before his death, but they had been "deaccessioned"—formally removed from the library's holdings— shortly before my visit to Kansas City. "Nobody has ever asked for them before—over thirty years," Dawn McInnis told me. She had intended to shred the papers, if only to free up valuable storage space, which was why the name rang a bell when Arlene contacted her.

"I hope it wasn't too much trouble," I said.

"Not at all," Dawn smiled. "I'm delighted that someone might find them useful." She pointed to a library cart holding ten large archival boxes. "I guess they've been waiting for you this whole time."

I rolled the cart over to a desk. Sutton had written several medical textbooks on dermatology and countless academic papers, apparently; hence the daunting amount of material before me. But fortunately, I was able to zero in on the papers related solely to *Sixteenth Century Physician*, packed in neatly labeled files. I found Miss Blasé's original typescript for *De excrementis*, along with a small trove of correspondence between Dr. Sutton and his translator.

Irene Blasé's translation—completed in 1966, their correspondence confirmed—did not look like a final draft. Every page of the chapter titled *De sudoribus* (Latin for sweat), thirty pages in length, was filled with her crossings-out, queries, alternate phrasings, and emendations. Even so, the essence of Mercuriale's thoughts and findings about sweat and sweating—all delivered in lectures transcribed by one of his medical students—was clear. Clearest of all (though not surprising, given how little was known at the time about the workings of the human body) was how wrong Mercuriale was—even absurdly wrong, it sometimes seemed. As with the *Gymnastica*, he was relying largely on the revered ancients of medicine and philosophy—Hippocrates, Galen, Plato, Avicenna, Diocles, Theophrastus, and others. Humoral theory; a belief in invisible substances that animated the body (*spiritus*) or emanated vaporously from it (*miasmas*); and, crucially, the long-standing prohibition against dissection of human cadavers kept these thinkers from seeing what now may seem obvious. Mercuriale was often reiterating the errors of his elders. To wit: "Sweat is nothing but a portion of potable substance changed in the liver [where blood was thought to be formulated], and transmitted naturally in the blood as a carrier through the veins, and finally expelled from the veins themselves through the hidden breathing." The "hidden breathing" was a sort of shortcut to explain the unexplainable, as I understand it, and provided just enough of a visual image to suffice, since the existence of sweat glands was then unknown. Exactly how sweat was excreted through the many "perforations"—pores—in the skin was not described in any detail.

The overall impression left by Mercuriale's writing in *De sudoribus*, however, was not how ridiculous his observations often were but instead how utterly mysterious—and therefore miraculous—the human body could be. And to be fair: Mercuriale did get a few things right. About the "substance" of sweat, he noted, "Some sweats are said to be of a thick consistency, others are considered to be thin. This differentia [or, 'feature' or 'property,' Miss Blasé inserted in the margin, searching for the right word in English] is recognized both by touch and by sight." (Here he was referring to the difference between sweat excreted from apocrine as opposed to eccrine glands.) "There are also differentiae from the gustatory property: sweats are said to be bitter, salty, or sharp. It should not seem strange to anyone that I set forth the tastes of sweat. Galen in his book *De symptomatum causis*, writes, 'Sweat sometimes flows over the face profusely and even of necessity enters the mouth and is tasted by the sick.'"

Mercuriale offered a number of reasons for *why* one sweats (the humors, digestion, or illnesses), but never recognized the aspect of thermoregulation. And he noted only in passing that "some sweat comes in running, some in walking about (promenading), some in the wrestling place (palestra) and [with] exercise." Sweat developed from movement, he went on to say, "because the veins are filled with spiritus; this spiritus, moved hither and thither, opens the mouths of the veins and through these expels the material of sweat."

What such vigorous movement and sweating could lead to in reality—thirst, or weight loss, for example, not to mention smelly armpits—he had almost nothing to say in *De excrementis*. But in a volume published six years later, as it turned out, Mercuriale elaborated. I would have known nothing about this had it not been for the tenacious Irene Blasé. To my astonishment, I found in one of the archival boxes an unlabeled file folder filled with yet another marked-up typescript on onion-skin paper: her complete translation of one of the most obscure and seemingly eccentric Mercuriale texts—his 1585 volume known as *De decoratione liber* (*The Book on Bodily Beauty*, or *Bodily Embellishment*, which included the doctor's views on the "art of cosmetics"). It took me a few minutes to put two and two together. This book, transcribed from another public lecture, is rarely mentioned in descriptions of Mercuriale's oeuvre (perhaps because it is viewed as so inconsequential in terms of serious scholarship), and I certainly never expected to find it on my visit to Kansas City. But there it was, all two hundred pages transmuted through Miss Blasé's words.

Like *De sudoribus*, none of *De decoratione* had ever been published in English; indeed, it is not clear why she went to all the effort to track down a copy of Mercuriale's original and translate it. Did Dr. Sutton commission her, as he had with *De morbis cutaneis*? Perhaps, though I found no evidence of this. He had paid her fairly for her work—five dollars per page—but that didn't seem to matter to her very much, comments in her correspondence suggested, nor did she wish for any credit in his publications.

"As you know, translation is a pleasant experience for me," Miss Blasé wrote to Dr. Sutton in a handwritten note, "more pleasant with a purpose than without." She was blind in one eye, had cataracts in her "good" eye, and seemed to have some orthopedic problems, but that didn't stop her. Simply put, she enjoyed it. "Whether I can do the translation is more a matter of logistics rather than linguistics. I do not sit comfortably at a table to work, but put my typewriter in my lap, while I sit in a recliner." I could picture Miss Blasé, absorbed for hours and days and weeks on end, with Mercuriale's text on one side and a "dictionary at hand," typing away as she tried to hear, from a distance of four hundred years, what this "very learned" doctor had to say.

"LET US BEGIN," Mercuriale says in his opening remarks for *De decoratione.* "The practitioner of the art of beauty care gives attention not only to preserving beauty, but also to removing ugliness, since this cannot be done without recognizing and removing those diseases which cause ugliness." Diseases and defects specifically of the skin—whether boils, acne, lice, infections, or other dermatological maladies—he had already addressed in *De morbis cutaneis*, he notes, whereas here he will discuss matters of appearance, size, and shape, the problem of "excessive size" being among the most serious. It goes by various names, he notes: "The Latins call it now corpulence, now obesity, now fatness . . . This condition or this blemish is great grossness of the whole body, damaging beauty and movement," for those who are "too fat" can scarcely walk, as if "held in a very massive prison." Among the causes: "Copious drinking of rich and excellent wine" and many "rich" foods, including eggs, pastries, bread, and sauces.

As for a cure, Mercuriale echoes Hippocrates: "He who wishes to be freed from obesity . . . must spoil leisure, [and] exercise as strenuously as possible . . . to the point when the breath is panting on account of effort." In short, Mercuriale recommends high-intensity cardiovascular training for weight loss. But he has another important recommendation: "Coitus especially reduces fat and flesh. Hence, it is apparent that all lustful animals for this reason are thin and emaciated, because the substance of fat and flesh is consumed in the practice of coitus."

I loved how straightforward he was about this. I thought it revealed something about him—that this respected and religious physician wasn't prudish about sex.

All of this sweaty physical activity, needless to say, could cause a "disagreeable odor" to arise, he noted. Although there was no special term in either Latin or Greek for smelly feet, he points out, there is one for the "bad odor from the armpits" caused by excess sweating: *goatiness*, in Miss Blasé's phrase (from the Latin *capra* or *caper* for goat). "Among the ancients the most ignominious condition was to smell as a goat," an odor so horrible "that sometimes it can scarcely be endured," Mercuriale adds. But the physician from Forli had several prescriptions for homemade deodorants. "If the fetor comes from the armpits, the kind which offends the noses of many, there are two ways to help. One is washing under the arms carefully with rose water, water of flowers of citron, fragrant wine, or alternatively aloe wood . . . If this method is not satisfactory, the other is to use substances whose odor will smother the odor of the armpits. The ancients . . . carried under their arms sometimes amomum [cardamom], sometimes myrrh, sometimes cinnamon." Ambergris would also do. As for himself, he finds that "aloes mixed with other perfumes can remove all underarm odors."

I gave my underarms a discreet sniff, and my Gillette Cool Wave deodorant suddenly seemed terribly prosaic. Next time I have some fragrant wine and flowers of citron nearby, I thought to myself, I might just have to try them instead.

The Art of Swimming

I plunged in, and bade him follow: so indeed he did.
The torrent roar'd; and we did buffet it with lusty sinews.

—WILLIAM SHAKESPEARE, *JULIUS CAESAR*, 1599

There is some question among scholars about whether Girolamo Mercuriale practiced what he preached—whether he himself exercised for the benefit of his health. If so, he never says so outright in the *Gymnastica*. But I believe clues come through between the lines. His description of swimming, for instance: Only someone who has swum would say, as he does, that "in the movement involved in swimming, the entire body is affected and put to work." He goes on to cite Aristotle, who observed that it was "not inappropriate" to compare swimming to running. And it's true, one could do a kind of head count of body parts and see that each one is engaged while swimming: eyes, mouth, nose, lungs, heart, shoulders, chest, arms, hands, neck, back, abdominal muscles, buttocks, legs, feet.

"Swimming can make one slender, improve the breath, firm up, warm and thin the body as well as rendering a person less liable to injury," Mercuriale pointed out. What's more, he felt that swimming provides "greater pleasure" than other kinds of exercise, "since the movement of the water . . . produces by its gentle touch a sort of peculiar pleasure all its own." Spoken like a true swimmer. I like that *peculiar pleasure*, how it acknowledges the frankly sensual nature of swimming and the relationship—if that's not too odd a word to use—that one develops with water. The environment in which the swimmer swims makes it unique among exercises, and uniquely satisfying.

But the water's embrace can change as quickly as the weather. As with fire, there is always an element of danger and unpredictability with water, whether one is swimming in a lake, river, ocean, pond, or pool, which puts swimming in a different category from other forms of exercise. This is not to say that risks are not inherent in running, lifting, climbing, cycling, martial arts, ball games, or yoga, but these tend to be injuries of overuse (pulled muscles, torn tendons), equipment failure, or perhaps an overzealous opponent (a boxer's black eye). And instances of so-called death by exercise—when someone drops dead while, say, jogging—are generally due to preexisting medical conditions (albeit often unknown) such as atrial fibrillation. With swimming, by contrast, your life depends on knowing how to do it. There can be a very real risk of drowning, of accidents occurring—being outmatched by a powerful current and carried out to sea, or taken under by a rogue wave—no matter how strong a swimmer you may be. Whereas parents teach their children to ride a bike for the sheer fun of it, for the sense of freedom and independence it brings, swimming is taught, first of all, as a basic safety measure. It's a parent's duty. The same was so thousands of years ago.

Our earliest recorded evidence of swimming comes in a group of cave paintings created during the Neolithic period, dating to about ten thousand years ago. The pictographs, found in a cave in southwest Egypt near the Libyan border, appear to show swimmers in different phases of a stroke—to my eyes, it looks like the breast-stroke. At the time these were painted, the climate was more temperate in this part of the world; there were lakes and rivers where now there is little more than desert. Archaeologists have postulated that the scenes depict an aspect of everyday life, a time when survival depended on knowing how to swim. One swam to reach the other side of a body of water—perhaps in pursuit of food, or to flee a warring tribe, or to move to safer ground—and one swam simply for sustenance: to catch fish.

Among the Greeks, it seems to have been expected that everyone—man, woman, and child—should be able to swim, which makes sense, since most people lived near the water. As Plato observes in the *Laws*, not knowing how to swim was considered as much a sign of ignorance as not knowing how to read. Socrates put it more starkly: Swimming "saves a man from death." Parents taught their children, and presumably children learned from one another. The same obligation has held true for many centuries in Judaism. As stated in the Talmud (Kiddishin 29a), parents must teach their children three essential things: the Torah, how to make a living, and how to swim.

A similar perspective held true in ancient Egypt, where most people lived on the Nile or on one of the canals branching from the river. The ability to swim was a life-and-death matter for fishermen or boatmen, and a mark of a proper education for the higher classes. In both Greece and Egypt, however, swimming was not among the events at athletic games or displays. (Swimming did not become an Olympic event until the advent of the modern games in 1896.) Exactly why this would be is never stated in ancient texts or hiero-glyphics, naturally—any more than we would feel compelled to justify today why walking or race-car driving isn't in the Olympics. My sense is that swimming was seen as more of a utilitarian skill—the "athletic equivalent of the alphabet," as the historian Christine

Nutton has put it—given that nearly everyone knew how to swim, women included, it fell outside an exclusively male sphere. Moreover, swimming was not a spectacular event, like ancient Greek or Roman boxing or pankration. And unlike sprints or field events, with their displays of speed and strength, it was not conducive to spectators. While swimming may not have been a competitive event, though, its value as an all-around exercise was apparently appreciated. Both the ancient historian Pausanias and the writer Philostratus noted that the four-time Olympic boxing champion Tisandrus supplemented his training at the gymnasium with long-distance swimming: in Philostratus's words, "his arms carried him great distances through the sea, training both his body and themselves."

Mastering swimming is a prerequisite for certain types of military service today, including, for obvious reasons, the U.S. Navy SEALs; this was more broadly the case in antiquity. In his treatise on military training, *De re militari*, Vegetius recommends, "Every young soldier, without exception, should in the summer months be taught to swim; for it is sometimes impossible to pass rivers on bridges, but the fleeing and pursuing army both are often obliged to swim over them. A sudden melting of snow or fall of rain often makes them overflow their banks, and in such a situation, the danger is as great from ignorance in swimming as from the enemy . . . The cavalry also as well as the infantry, and even the horses and the servants of the army should be accustomed to this exercise, as they are all equally liable to the same accidents."

Vegetius's treatise was translated into Italian, French, and German during the Renaissance and exerted influence on the training of the military and nobility up through the nineteenth century. In *The Book of the Courtier*, Baldesar Castiglione endorses the importance of swimming for a gentleman, citing Vegetius for backup. However, neither author explains *how* to swim. Actual instruction manuals on swimming didn't begin to appear until the sixteenth century.

The first of these, a stilted dialogue in praise of swimming titled *Colymbetes* and written in Latin by the Swiss humanist Nicolas Wyman, predated Mercuriale's *Gymnastica* by three decades. Wyman was concerned with teaching rescue techniques—holding on to the victim while swimming with the free arm. It was not until fifty years later, in 1587, that the Englishman Everard Digby would treat the topic fully in *De arte natandi* (*The Art of Swimming*). Digby, neither a physician nor an athlete per se, had been inspired by the work of a fellow scholar at St. John's College, Cambridge, the poet and teacher Roger Ascham. Ascham's 1545 treatise on archery, *Toxophilus* (*Lover of the Bow*), was the first of its kind—a step-by-step guide to shooting the longbow that also aspired to be a work of literary merit, written not in Latin but in plain English. As Ascham pointed out in prefatory remarks, "Many English writers have not done so, but using strange words, as Latin, French, and Italian, do make all things dark and hard." The book was dedicated to King Henry VII, who showed his approval by granting Ascham a yearly pension for life.

While Digby modeled his work on Ascham's, focusing on a single form of exercise, he persisted in making things "dark and hard" and inaccessible by writing in a scholar's Latin. Nearly a decade later, the poet Christopher Middleton translated Digby's *De arte natandi* into English; this version—reprinted numerous times and also translated into French—would remain the standard text on swimming in the Western world for another three hundred years. All things considered, it's not bad; it goes beyond Wyman's lifesaving techniques and makes a case for swimming as an art and a science well worth studying. Instructions are included for a breaststroke, dog paddle, treading water, and so on. (The freestyle stroke swum today would not be refined until the nineteenth century.) If anything, Digby goes too far, gets too imaginative. For instance, he recommends a kind of pedicure-cum-backstroke that sounds as ludicrous as it does dangerous. Speaking of a hypothetical student, he writes (in Middleton's translation): "Swimming upon his backe, let him draw up his left foote, and laye it over his right knee, still keeping his body very straight, and than hauing a knife ready in his right hand, he may easily keep up his legge until he hath pared one of his toes, as thus." One has to wonder if Digby actually tried this, or even swam at all.

I WAS TAUGHT how to swim at a big public pool in the park just down the block from our house in Spokane—I took the requisite Red Cross classes—but I'd say I really learned how to swim from my dad, former West Point swim team captain that he was. He'd been a competitive swimmer in high school, too, and never lost his love for the water. He passed his enthusiasm on to my sisters and me. We weren't a family that packed up the station wagon and took summer road trips to the Grand Canyon or Mount Rushmore or the Hoover Dam. We'd go boating at one of the nearby lakes in northern Idaho on weekends. Sometimes my best friend, Chris, came along. Dad didn't fish, and never sailed—too slow and boring for him. He liked speed. We had a motorboat with an Evinrude outboard—it was about fifteen feet long—and once he got the boat into the water and started (often an ordeal) he would floor it and we'd fly across the water. He'd kill the engine in the middle of the lake, pull out water skis and a towrope, and each of us would take a spin. My sisters and I had all known how to water-ski from a young age; we had to, whether we wanted to or not. By the time each of us was in high school, we had made the transition, under his tutelage, from two skis to slalom.

For a few weeks every summer, we rented a cabin at Priest Lake, just ninety minutes or so from Spokane. It's a deep and enormous lake—fifteen miles long—far larger than the many small lakes in Minnesota, where both my parents were born and raised. Dad would work all week at the Coke plant—summers were the busiest time of year for the soda pop business—and come out on weekends. Upon waking each morning, he'd go directly to the dock and without so much as a pause dive in. It seemed an impossibly long time before he'd surface—way beyond the buoy marking the deep end. Floating on his back, he'd shoot sprays of water through the gap in his front teeth. "Best way to start the day!" Dad would say after doing a vigorous butterfly back to the dock.

ONCE A YEAR, I join a group of friends I've known since high school for a long weekend at a cabin on the same lake, Priest Lake. We started this tradition the year after my partner Steve died in 2006—a way to come together other than at memorials and funerals, which become more frequent as the years go by. We hang out on the dock and drink beer and laugh and swim and catch up and, when evening comes, make cocktail shakers of margaritas and big meals together. We're back on the dock at night, stargazing, and talking about our lives, and drinking one or two more than we normally would. It's just a short walk back to the cabin; no harm done. When morning comes, I do exactly as my dad—a Scotch-and-soda guy—would do forty years ago: head for the lake and a quick, brisk morning swim. Nothing clears my head, gets my heart racing and blood pumping, and makes me feel more alive than sprinting through the water as fast as I can. By the time I'm out, someone has brought down a big pot of coffee, and the day starts all over again.

Except for these annual summer weekends at Priest Lake, though, I rarely swam during the other fifty-one weeks of the year. In fact, I hadn't swum much since college. I never belonged to a gym with a lap pool, and I suppose I'd forgotten how much I enjoyed swimming as a kid, how effortless it had once been. I discovered this was no longer so when, with Oliver's encouragement, I decided to take up swimming again in 2012. I joined a new gym with a twenty-five-meter pool. Getting back into the water and trying to do laps at age fifty-one was humbling. The first time, I couldn't do more than two without having to stop, badly winded. It's not that I wasn't "fit," but swimming is a cardiovascular workout unlike climbing a StairMaster or running on a treadmill. Being strong and muscular isn't enough; indeed, it can hamper one's ability because flexibility in the limbs is key. Swimming puts great demands on the whole body and makes the very act of breathing more challenging, more exhausting, than on land.

But I kept at it and began joining Oliver at the pool a couple of times a week. Because of my bad left shoulder, I couldn't comfortably do the backstroke or butterfly without strain, and the breaststroke had always seemed, unfairly perhaps, like the ultimate "B" stroke to me. I wanted to learn to do a good freestyle. So I watched videos on YouTube, and I studied a recent instructional book on swimming, Terry Laughlin's *Total Immersion*, which contained tips that helped: keep your head down, literally press it into the water, for instance (this helps keep your legs from dragging, too), and don't just turn your face to take a breath, rotate your whole body. But the most important factor was going back to the pool repeatedly. Swimming is a skill, a complex motor skill that has to be learned, or at my age relearned, and one can't skip the practice step in learning. It's like boxing in this way—the sometimes tedious process of struggling through to the point of greater mastery.

Almost by definition, practice involves making errors, recognizing them, and exploring ways to correct them, to make adjustments. I came to see that practicing is a phase distinct from exercising, though of course one "gets exercise" while practicing. Practice takes thought. At its best, its most satisfying, exercise does not. The moment one stops thinking about what one is doing—the kick, the stroke, the bilateral breathing—and just *does* it, the pleasure part of exercise begins.

Mercuriale had likened swimming to running, but I came to see this as a limited comparison. Running doesn't involve the upper body in a similar way. With the freestyle, I noticed how it feels more like a climb, a horizontal climb, across the surface of a body of water. (No wonder it's also called the crawl.) One is grabbing handfuls of water, as if on the face of a cliff, and pulling oneself forward—I pictured myself as Spider-Man scampering up a building. The water operates as a force of resistance against which one's muscles are working. The torso, powered by the hips and buttocks, rotates rapidly, causing the body to churn through the water like a giant industrial drill tunneling through rock face.

The more I swam, the more I enjoyed using my body as a means of transportation, getting from one side of the pool to the other in a matter of seconds; in this way, it did resemble running (or, flying). I bought short fins so I could swim even faster. I would time my fifty-meter laps and try to shave off a second. By the time I returned to Priest Lake for our annual reunion, I had become a more confident swimmer. Instead of a quick dip, I would put on my goggles and fins and swim along the shore to docks four or five cabins down the lake, a half mile or so and back. I swam several times a day.

On our last day, after half our group had left to return home, four of us took the boating equivalent of a road trip to Upper Priest Lake—a remote, wild, almost untouched part of northern Idaho just a few miles from the Canadian border—where we hiked and had a picnic. The boat ride back to the cabin was long; by the time we returned, it was 3:40 in the afternoon. I know this precisely because when we were pulling into the dock, one of us, I think it was me, asked what time it was.

My friend Chris's wife, Shannon, looked at her watch and said, "Three forty."

We all took this in, nodding and calculating in our heads what we had time for, what we needed to do, before leaving the cabin for the drive back to Spokane. It had been a glorious, almost magical day and we had gotten back later than originally planned. There were bags to be packed, beds to be stripped, the cabin to be cleaned, cars loaded. But first things first: We were all scorching hot and thirsty from the long boat ride on a cloudless ninety-two-degree day, and frankly, we all had to use a bathroom.

Melaine and I hopped out of the boat as Chris pulled into the dock; we secured the boat and gathered up our belongings. I remember Chris saying he "really, really" had to take a piss, and seeing him heading up to the cabin, almost running. It passed through my mind to do the same but then I thought better of it: *I want to swim anyway, so I'll just take a leak in the lake.* Shannon and Melaine were already in the water. I sat on the dock for a moment. I didn't have my swim goggles with me and I thought about getting them from my bag. "Nah," I told myself. So I plopped into the water, took a deep breath, and shoved off swimming underwater.

My legs are strong. When I push off, my body is streamlined, arms stretched out before me in a V. With some good speed behind me, I took two, if not three, full breaststrokes under water. I loved doing these—the gliding feeling, as if I were a manta ray skimming the lake bottom—especially when I'd pull my hands back all the way to my sides before starting another stroke. I still remember that lovely gliding, arms tucked tight, and then—*bang*, a single, loud clanking in my head—and the instant sensation that there'd been a terrible mistake. It was like hearing music that is suddenly cut off by ugly distortion, or seeing a computer screen suddenly go blank. I surfaced, and instinctively turned toward the dock and heard myself saying in a loud voice, "I hit a rock. I hit a rock . . . !"

I want them to know. That's what was going through my head: It's important that they know, that I say what happened. My head was ringing, and I thought I might pass out. I knew it was bad; I heard that sound. Yet I also found myself calmly walking toward the dock in the chest-high water, as I heard Shannon and Melaine gasping as they watched me coming toward them with blood running down my face.

I don't know exactly how far out I had been—maybe twenty-five meters, a pool's length, I'm not sure—yet far enough that the large rock I'd hit on the bottom of the lake was not something one could have seen from shore.

I reached the dock, and Melaine, a medical technician at a Spokane hospital, was already coming toward me with a beach towel, which she dropped onto my head, telling me to push hard on the cut. One of the two said something about all the blood, the blood in my beard. Melaine kept repeating to press down on the cut. I was telling myself to breathe. I had one hand on the dock, one on my forehead. I stood there for a couple of seconds, and then I heard Melaine say something like, "We have to figure out how to get you out of the water." I didn't answer; I just hoisted myself onto the dock with my free hand. I stood up, someone said, "Sit down, sit down." Shannon got a lawn chair and put it under me.

I was dazed. I knew something bad had happened. I'd had an accident—not "I was in an accident" or "it was an accident," neither of which imply any fault on one's part, but "I had an accident." Something about this phrase, going through my head, immediately said to me that it had been my fault. It was I, I, I who had done it. The accident was my fault. If only I had worn my goggles, if only I had swum with eyes open, if only I had gone up to the cabin to use the bathroom, if only I hadn't been in a hurry.

By now, Chris was back from the cabin, and he and Melaine said they were going to take a look at the cut. Shannon again said something about the blood—"there are a lot of blood vessels in the head," she said a few times. But I remained calm and tried to focus on breathing. They asked if I was cold. "No." They asked if I wanted water.

"Yes." I kept pressing and did as I was told. Melaine zoomed into my range of vision as she carefully pulled back the towel and peeked. Her face was serious and concerned. She nodded. "You're going to be okay," she said, but her expression wasn't quite so reassuring.

Chris left and came back a while later—it seemed like a long time—with butterfly bandages. (His dad is a doctor, and they had a complete first aid kit in the cabin.) Everyone was saying things, and I was just lost in my head. Eventually, Chris opened a bandage, Shannon sprayed Neosporin on it, Melaine peeled off the towel, and Chris placed two butterfly bandages, tightly sealing the gash. They put the towel back and told me to keep pressing on the cut. By this point, I had to pee so bad I felt that I couldn't even remember how to pee, but sitting there on the dock didn't seem to be a good idea, so I stood up and walked with the three of them to the cabin. I would go see a doctor back in Spokane.

I locked the door behind me in the bathroom and took a look in the mirror. Dried blood crusted my forehead and beard. I could see through the two butterfly bandages that the gash on my forehead was about the length of my thumb, about two inches, right under the hairline. The skin around it was scraped. I splashed water on my face and cleaned my beard and finally sat down on the toilet and emptied my bladder, and then I just sat there for a long while. A conversation came back to me. I remembered once talking to an older fellow at the gym, a former bodybuilder, after I learned I had a torn rotator cuff tendon. I was feeling discouraged. He told me he had had the same thing happen to him but that, if I did physical therapy and gave it a rest, I would be okay. "It's gonna go away," he said. "It'll just be part of your history."

I liked that. I liked putting the injury in that context. The accident, my accident, could have killed me, or left me paralyzed, or with a fracture. I could have drowned, if I'd been alone. I was still shaken by this, and I had a kind of sickening feeling knowing that the memory of hitting that rock—that *clank* sound, the burst of distortion in my brain—would probably be with me for a long time. The scar that would form on my forehead would mark this one particular moment in my life. It has since shrunk over time, so that it's far less visible, but the fear it put into me about the danger of swimming in unfamiliar waters remains. And from that day on, I have never swum without wearing goggles.

Inside the Archive

The only possible form of exercise is to talk, not to walk.

—OSCAR WILDE (1854–1900)

Monsieur Agasse had seen with his own eyes and held with his own hands countless letters from and to Mercuriale, codices of lectures transcribed by his devoted students, and rare first editions of Mercuriale's books, all of which Agasse—being a Latin scholar—could read in the original language. But one thing, he admitted with a sigh of regret when we had met in Paris, had proved frustratingly elusive: He had never been able to examine firsthand the surviving original drawings done by Pirro Ligorio for *De arte gymnastica*. The drawings are held in the private collection of one of the oldest and wealthiest families in Italy, the Borromeo family. Agasse had tried numerous times to gain access but with no luck.

By that point, my own attempts to contact members of the family, their representatives, or staff at the archive had been equally fruitless, partly because I was not fluent in Italian, I presumed, so I took a different approach. I found an Italian-language translator to do some reconnaissance for me. This fellow—Giovanni was his name—lived near Forlì, Mercuriale's hometown. After doing some digging, he reported back to me:

> Dear Mr. Hayes,
>
> I managed to contact an official of the Sovrintendenza Archivistica della Lombardia in Milan (Archive and Heritage Department of Lombardy), who lectured me about the rise and fall of the original Archivio Borromeo, how its documents are now to be found in a number of different archives, among which are the Archivio Borromeo d'Adda, the Archivio Litta Visconti Borromeo Arese, and the Archivio Borromeo d'Isola Bella. On the first two, nothing matches your request. As for the latter, he could not do much for me, he regretted, as this does not fall under the Sovrintendenza Archivistica della Lombardia, but under the Sovrintendenza Archivistica del Piemonte (Piedmont) in Turin. The point of contact there is Mrs. Esilda Manuguerra.

My exceedingly polite letter to Mrs. Esilda Manuguerra went unanswered, so, short of giving up, I made an inquiry with the Italian publisher of the *Gymnastica*, asking for suggestions. It was so obvious, I should have thought of this sooner. In a matter of days, I received word that I had been given permission to visit the Archivio Borromeo d'Isola Bella—but only at a very specific time and date: eleven A.M. on a Sunday in November, less than a month away. I was told there was no flexibility on this.

I hardly thought twice; I booked a flight to Milan.

A year and a half after my visits to London and Paris, I took a red-eye from New York, dropped my bags at a cheap hotel near the Milan train station, and took a train to Stresa, a small town near the Italian-Swiss border on Lake Maggiore. Following the directions

I had been given, I exited the train station, took a right, then a left down an empty, winding street toward the lake, where I found a small, makeshift ticket booth for a ferry. Tourist season was long over; there was hardly anyone else in sight. But within minutes, a motorboat pulled up to a small, portable dock positioned on the beach. Six other passengers were already on board. I scampered across the rickety structure, as if walking a plank in a dream. Morning fog clinging to the water obscured any view of where we were headed. The boat made stops at three small islands on Lake Maggiore, and couple by couple, all the other passengers disappeared.

At last, my turn came. "Ecco la," the ferryboat captain said, with a wave of his hand. I hopped out and the boat roared away. It was 10:55, the fog had dissipated, and I found myself standing on the shore of a place that could not possibly have been more aptly named: La Isola Bella—Beautiful Island. Rising against a picture-postcard backdrop of snowcapped mountains meeting the deep blue lake was what looked like an enchanted castle—the baroque-era Palazzo Borromeo.

How does one say *speechless* in Italian?

That was one of the first questions I asked my host, a genial, dimpled fellow in his early fifties, who found me in a jetlagged daze not far from the dock.

"Senza parole," he answered, after introducing himself. His name was Alessandro, but he told me to call him Alex.

"Senza parole, yes, senza parole . . ."

Before visiting the archive, Alex suggested that we stop for a coffee. Isola Bella is dominated by the enormous Borromeo palazzo and gardens, yet other people do live on the tiny island year-round, and there were a few small shops and cafés open. Alex ordered espressos and an almost comically large slice of chocolate cake to share. His English was good enough that we were easily able to begin getting acquainted.

It took me a while to put two and two together, but eventually it dawned on me why I hadn't been able to locate an office, email address, or any other contact info for the Archivio Borromeo: There was no office. There was no full-time archivist. There was no staff as such. What there was, simply and solely, was one man—the man sitting across from me, finishing off a piece of chocolate cake—who happened to be the devoted son of the former professional archivist for the Borromeo family. Alex's father died suddenly in 1991, and since that day Alex had done his best to carry on his father's legacy. He worked full-time as an engineer during the week off the island, in a town ninety miles from there, and, since he reserved Saturdays for his wife and kids, could only come to Isola Bella on some Sundays to take care of business. The Borromeo family preferred not to hire anyone else to tend to the archive, and Alex rarely heard from them. It was Alex alone who held the key.

And what a key it was: a large, old-fashioned pewter key. It looked like it was forged for a medieval jail cell. Alex led me into the palazzo, through a series of grand and elegantly appointed rooms, all empty, and finally ushered me into a circular salon that opened onto the Hall of Tapestries, lined with astonishing works from as early as the fourteenth century. I would have lingered there, but Alex called me over. Almost hidden in the salon's wall was a tall narrow door, which he opened with the giant pewter key.

I followed Alex through it, up a winding flight of steep stairs, and into a small dark room that could have been mistaken for a storage closet. Even so, there was protocol to follow: I had to first sign in, just as I did each time I visited the Rare Books room at the Academy of Medicine, although this registry went back over a century.

Alex mentioned that I was in good company: "Mr. Ernest Hemingway" signed the book on a visit to the Palazzo Borromeo in September 1918. Alex found the entry and showed me Hemingway's signature. I was incredulous, but I realized that Hemingway—long before he was *Hemingway*—enlisted as an ambulance driver with the Red Cross and was sent to Italy early that same year; he was all of eighteen. Just a month into his service, he was badly wounded and spent some six months in a rehab hospital in Milan. It was plausible that he too had made a day trip to Lake Maggiore.

Alex cleared space from a broad table and placed on it a folio resembling an oversized manila folder. "Allora," he said, and gestured toward it, inviting me to proceed.

"The drawings? These are the drawings?" I had imagined the precious, nearly five-hundred-year-old Ligorio works would be framed, hung on a wall.

Alex smiled his boyish smile. "Sì, the drawings," he said.

IT WOULD BE difficult to imagine the *Gymnastica* surviving or succeeding—going into multiple editions and translations—without those drawings. I certainly wouldn't have been there if not for the spell they had cast. If, say, Ms. Shaner had brought out the unillustrated 1569 edition instead, I might have leafed through the impenetrable Latin text, closed the book, and not given it another thought. But I have begun to think that Pirro Ligorio may have played an even bigger role than he is given credit for. Although his images did not appear until the second edition, published in 1573, I had a hunch that Ligorio may have planted a seed—if not *the* seed—for the book in Mercuriale's mind in the first place. After all, it's never been entirely clear or obvious why Mercuriale would take on such a project. He wasn't predisposed to do so, other than knowing Latin and Greek. The only clue Mercuriale provided was that the ruins of ancient Roman thermal baths and gymnasia—the Baths of Caracalla, of Diocletian, and others—had inspired him. But these were not the tourist sights they are today, complete with explanatory texts, and in fact were still largely unexcavated when Mercuriale lived in Rome. One would have to know about them, be *shown* them, and few were more knowledgeable about these buildings and their history, or more passionate about their significance, than Pirro Ligorio.

We know the two men met soon after Mercuriale arrived in Rome. At the time, Ligorio served both as a superintendent of the ancient monuments and as architect of the Vatican Palace, under Pope Pius IV. More so than Mercuriale, he was truly a Renaissance man—a painter, writer, architect, archaeologist, cartographer, and antiquarian scholar. He was in close contact with the Farnese librarians Fulvio Orsini and Onofrio Panvinio, who had assisted Ligorio in a monumental project to re-create a map of ancient Rome—a "labor of love," in Ligorio's words, which had been published the year before. As the historian Howard Burns has noted, "It was a work which condensed the results of more than two decades of intensive research and writing [by Ligorio], and it could not have been achieved in its final form without reference to the massive corpus of antiquarian writings and thousands of drawings of ancient buildings, coins, inscriptions, and reliefs, which Ligorio had by this time built up." He had already published smaller maps of ancient Rome as well as engravings of the Baths of Diocletian, the Circus Maximus—the primary venue for chariot races and gladiatorial games—and other ancient sites. A prolific writer, he had also begun work on his unprecedented, if highly eccentric, "encyclopedia of antiquarianism," a project that would run to thirty volumes by the time of his death (yet still be unfinished and unpublished). It's not inconceivable that Ligorio himself could have written a book on the ancient art of exercise, albeit not from the specialized perspective of a physician. In any case, whereas Mercuriale had time to devote to such a book, Ligorio had his hands more than full with numerous architectural projects, including a revised design for the Belvedere Courtyard, a summer house for Pius IV, and a small palazzo in Rome for the pope. Perhaps his most illustrious commission, however, was to succeed Michelangelo as architect for the completion of St. Peter's Basilica in 1564—apparently beating out the great artist in an architectural competition.

However, things soon began to go south for Ligorio.

For reasons not entirely clear, he was accused of larceny (falsely, apparently) and put in prison. (One has to wonder if his perceived rival, Michelangelo, might have had something to do with this, even tangentially.) Ligorio implored Cardinal Farnese to intercede on his behalf, and he was finally released without further charges after three weeks. Now in his midfifties, Ligorio managed to continue on in Rome for a time. But he ran into further trouble upon publicly criticizing Michelangelo's work in St. Peter's and was subsequently fired by the pope. To make ends meet, he sold his collection of medals to Cardinal Farnese, but it must have been clear that he had become persona non grata in Rome. Once again, the cardinal seems to have pulled some strings. Ligorio was appointed "antiquarian" in the court of Duke Alfonso II d'Este, one of Farnese's nephews; this was quite a step down from being architect of the Vatican as well as one of the most sought-after artists, but at least this was a stable position and guaranteed income. He had five children to support. He moved to the duke's court in Ferrara right around the time that the first edition of Mercuriale's book came out.

How things had changed! Whereas Ligorio was lucky to have a job at all, Mercuriale's star was rising. The first edition of *De arte gymnastica* was successful enough to encourage Mercuriale to begin work on a revised edition for which his publisher agreed to pay for engraved illustrations—something that would make the book even more distinctive and appealing. After all, they had had success publishing illustrated manuals on medicine, anatomy, and religion. Pictures helped sell books. As luck would have it, his talented former colleague Pirro Ligorio was now living not far away.

ALEX OPENED THE folio. The first drawing was completely unfamiliar to me: an image of two men engaged in combat, one holding a trident and a large net, the other clutching what looked like a giant mallet overhead.

"Someone's going to die here," I commented. "Gladiators?"

Alex nodded vigorously. What it portrayed was a specific type of contest involving *retiarii*, or "net men"—sort of a combination of bullfighting and spearfishing, minus a bull or fish. Alex explained that this was one drawing, presumably the only one, that Mercuriale chose to leave out of the *Gymnastica*—a smart move on his part, as it might have invited scrutiny by church authorities, given the ban on duels by the Council of Trent. Even so, it was interesting to me that Ligorio should have even drawn it, for it marked that fascinating footnote in the history of exercise—the beginning of the end of athletics when the Roman emperor Constantine banned gladiatorial contests in A.D. 325.

Alex apologized for not having a better table, better lighting, better conditions, yet he encouraged me to take my time in examining the drawings. "Do it yourself—you can rejoice in the handling of it," he put it in his exuberant way.

I carefully went through the drawings—the wrestlers, boxers, the men with weights, rope climbers, and women on a swing. The paper was fragile, brittle, somewhat yellowed, but the drawings were in good condition. I could hardly believe my good fortune. "It's like touching Ligorio and, almost, as if I'm meeting Mercuriale," I whispered, "touching history—"

"—Sì, sì! Come sei dice complice?"

My face was a blank.

Alex struggled to come up with comparable words in English. Frustrated, he exclaimed, "Aspetta! Complice, complice," murmuring to himself.

"Friendship?" I try.

"No, no, no, no . . . What is it when you do something for instance during a robbery? I go with a gun, and you stay with me, but you don't participate with the gun yourself, but you stay nearby. You are—"

"On the lookout? Watching for the police?" I didn't have the faintest idea what this had to do with Ligorio and Mercuriale, or with Alex and me.

"No, no, no, when you're as I am. When I kill someone, you are . . . helping me, but you're on the side . . . You're?"

"Oh! An accomplice?"

"Sì! Sì! Sì! An accomplice!"

Thank God, I felt my head was about to explode.

"Accomplice. *Complicit*," he clarified. "I would like to establish a sort of complicity between us, so this way, more people will know about Ligorio and the archive."

"Absolutely," I told him. We shook hands.

Now, a conspiratorial smile came over his face. "Let me show you something," Alex said, "the drawing of the boxers."

I reached for the image of two men fighting, each with an arm upraised.

"No, not that, the other one, this one," Alex said, pointing to Ligorio's close-up of two boxers' hands, each wrapped in studded leather straps. "Do you notice anything different about this?"

I pointed out that this was surely not realistic—boxers didn't wear metal-studded straps like this, essentially the equivalent of brass knuckles. Ligorio took liberties here, as he did elsewhere. (Although he claimed that the images were authentic re-creations, based on ancient coins, that was not true.) But this was not what Alex had in mind. He told me to count the fingers on each hand.

"One, two, three, four, five, six—six, seven?" The thumb was clear, but the fingers, all six or seven of them, were out of proportion. I grabbed my copy of the *Gymnastica* and found the illustration of the boxers' hands. Where Ligorio's lines were loose and sketchy, the block cutter's were distinct, clean, well defined. It was as if Ligorio literally provided a quick sketch, not bothering to get it anatomically right, a rough draft that the printer's craftsmen finalized in the elaborate process of transforming the drawing into an illustration. (This was done by transferring Ligorio's drawing to a block of wood, then carving away everything not meant to be printed, leaving a relief surface to carry the printer's ink.) Seeing the before and after of this illustration brought out two things: how swiftly Ligorio must have drawn the image—it may have taken him no more than a few minutes, by the looks of it—and how credit for their visual impact, their boldness, their punch, must go equally to the craftsmen who made the woodcuts yet went uncredited, as was the custom.

"How could he make that mistake?" Alex wondered.

"Fastidiousness was not really in his nature," I responded. Ligorio was a man in a hurry, constantly juggling projects, trying to make ends meet. But at least Ferrara proved to be a stable place for him. Ten years after completing the drawings for Mercuriale, he would die there, age seventy, leaving his wife and children practically penniless. In the meantime, he had completed one major project that survives today: ceiling frescoes for the duke at his castle, undertaken after a terrible earthquake had destroyed much of the original building. I had heard that the frescoes were based on either his drawings for Mercuriale's *Gymnastica* or the other way around— that the drawings had been copied from the fresco images. It wasn't clear which came first. Alex said that he had never visited the castle and urged me to go, though not just to see the Ligorio frescoes.

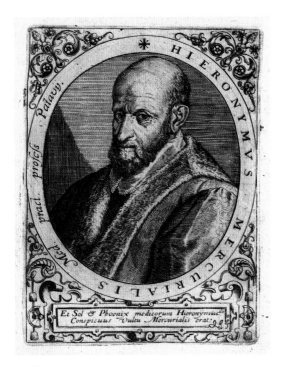

Girolamo Mercuriale (Hieronymus Mercurialis), author of *De arte gymnastica*, the first comprehensive, illustrated book on exercise; copper engraving by Johann Theodor de Bry, ca. 1598. COLLECTION OF THE RIJKS MUSEUM, AMSTERDAM

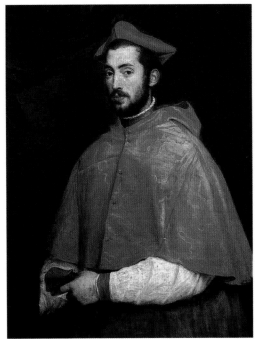

Cardinal Alessandro Farnese, by Titian, ca. 1545–1546. COLLECTION OF NATIONAL MUSEUM OF CAPODIMONTE, NAPLES, ITALY

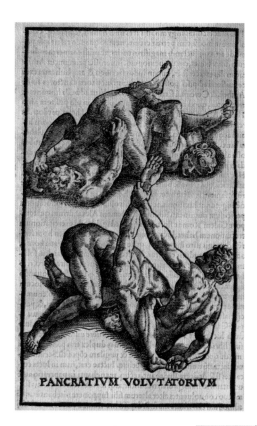

PANCRATIVM VOLVTATORIVM

Wrestlers, by Pirro Ligorio, from Mercuriale's *De arte gymnastica,* 1573. PHOTOGRAPH BY THE AUTHOR; COLLECTION OF THE SWEDISH SCHOOL OF SPORT AND HEALTH SCIENCES, GIH

Plan for a gymnasium based on the writings of Vitruvius, from Mercuriale's *De arte gymnastica,* 1569 edition.
PHOTOGRAPH BY THE AUTHOR; COLLECTION OF THE SWEDISH SCHOOL OF SPORT AND HEALTH SCIENCES, GIH, STOCKHOLM

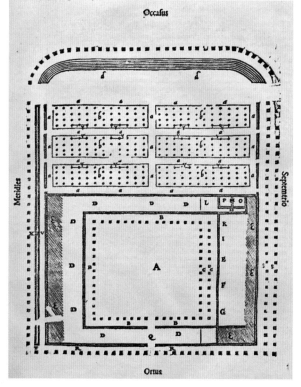

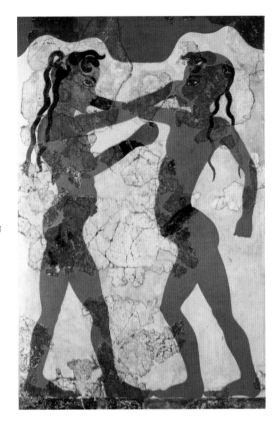

Akrotiri Boxer Fresco, ca. 1700 B.C. One of the earliest representations of athletics, the "Boxing Boys" were painted on the walls of an ancient Theran palace on what is now the island of Santorini. COLLECTION OF NATIONAL ARCHAEOLOGICAL MUSEUM, ATHENS

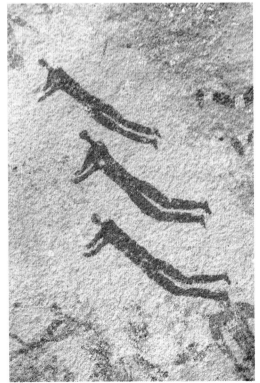

Painted figures from "Cave of the Swimmers," Mestekawi Cave, Gilf Kebir, Western Desert, Egypt, ca. 9,000 B.C.; one of the earliest representations of swimming.

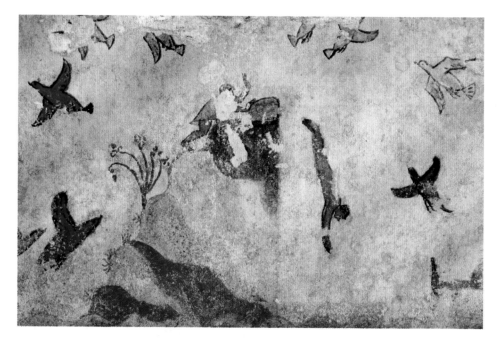

Diver in the Etruscan "Tomb of Hunting and Fishing," Tarquinia, Italy, ca. sixth century B.C. Archaeologists believe that scenes such as this depict an aspect of everyday life, at a time when survival depended on knowing how to swim.

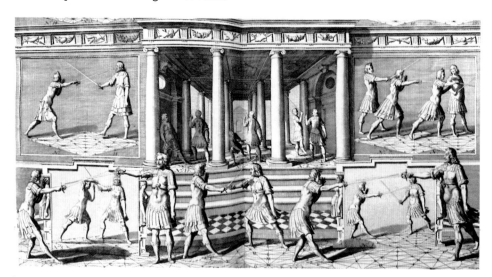

Academie de l'Espée, by Gérard Thibault d'Anvers, 1630; one of the most elaborate illustrated books on the art of fencing. PHOTOGRAPH BY THE AUTHOR; COLLECTION OF THE SWEDISH SCHOOL OF SPORT AND HEALTH SCIENCES, GIH, STOCKHOLM

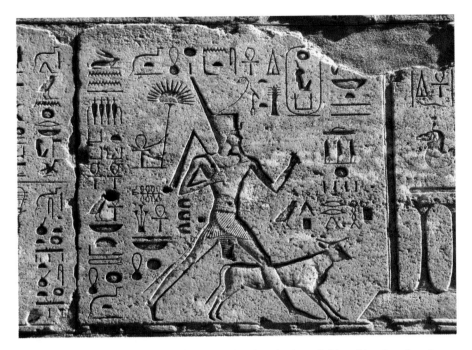

Wall relief of Queen Hatshepsut (one of the first female pharaohs) in a "ritual run" at the Heb-Sed festival, Eighteenth Dynasty, Egypt (ca. 1479–1458 B.C.); one of the earliest known representations of a human being running, not for the purpose of hunting or survival but as an act of homage to their gods.

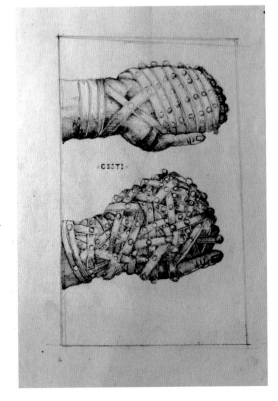

Caestus, original drawing of boxers' wrapped hands, by Pirro Ligorio, for Mercuriale's *De arte gymnastica*, 1573 edition. PHOTOGRAPH BY THE AUTHOR; COURTESY OF ARCHIVIO BORROMEO, L'ISOLA BELLA, ITALY, AND THE BORROMEO ARESE FAMILY

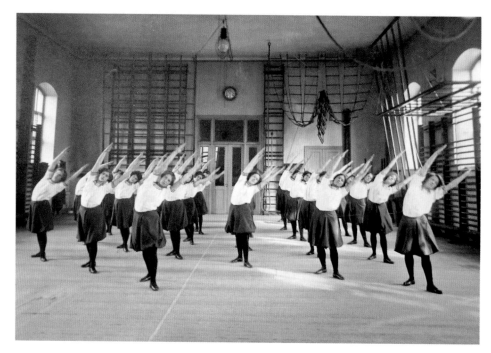

Class at the Royal Central Institute of Gymnastics, Stockholm, ca. 1890. Founded by Pehr Henrik Ling in 1813, the school was the first in the world devoted solely to the teaching and training of physical education—for men and women alike. COLLECTION OF THE SWEDISH SCHOOL OF SPORT AND HEALTH SCIENCES, GIH, STOCKHOLM

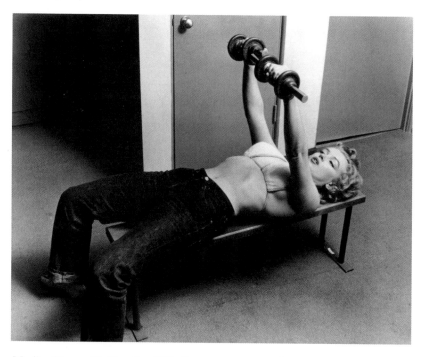

Marilyn Monroe Working Out, 1952. ©PHILIPPE HALSMAN/MAGNUM PHOTOS

Swami Vivekananda, an influential yogi who traveled and lectured widely in the United States, and established yoga centers around the world, ca. 1885–1895, at Jaipur.

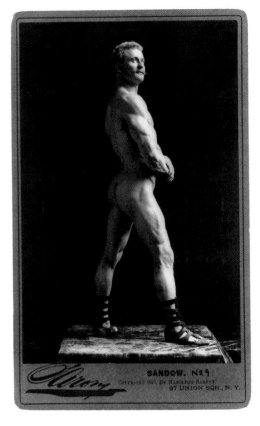

Eugen Sandow, photograph by Napoleon Sarony, 1893. A Prussian-born bodybuilder who found international fame for his "perfect" physique, Sandow published numerous books outlining his weightlifting and exercise regime, toured America and India, and opened fitness gyms under his name.

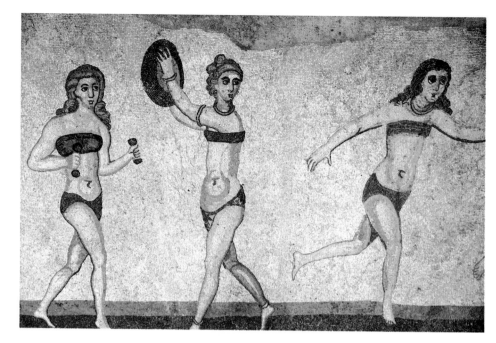

Floor mosaic of women engaging in sports, aka "Bikini Girls Mosaic," Villa Romana del Casale, Piazza Armerina, Sicily, A.D. fourth century; a UNESCO World Heritage Site.

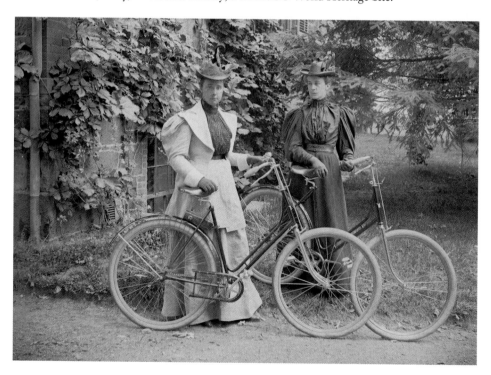

Violet Ward and Daisy Elliott with Bicycles, glass plate negative, by Alice Austen, ca. 1895. COLLECTION OF HISTORIC RICHMOND TOWN

"You can't go to Ferrara without tasting the sugo and the Bolognese," he said, adding wistfully, "you cannot imagine how much I love food."

I laughed. "Speaking of which, I'm starving—let's go eat. Can I treat you to lunch?"

"Certamente," said the guardian of Ligorio's drawing.

A Refutation of Those Who Think Everyone Should Exercise

Not less than two hours a day should be devoted to exercise, and the weather shall be little regarded. If the body is feeble, the mind will not be strong.

—THOMAS JEFFERSON (1743–1826)

I had been in Italy for three days and seen exactly one person exercising: a young man jogging through the cobblestone streets of Padua on the night I arrived from Milan (quite possibly an American, if an NYU T-shirt and a look of grim determination were any indication). I tracked down one gym as I wandered around and found it empty. Instead, I saw young couples kissing; men gathered smoking; students in clusters arguing and laughing; and bicyclists, scores of them, riding chiefly for transportation, it seemed. Hardly any cars were in this small, cloistered city, just bicycles—the soft whirring of their wheels the only sound other than the softly falling rain—bicyclists steering with the right hand, holding an umbrella with the other, so easily, as if that were exactly what a left hand is for.

Naturally, I wondered what Mercuriale would have made of this—bicycles! (Claims that Leonardo da Vinci designed a bicycle have proved untrue. It was not invented until the nineteenth century.) The doctor would have approved, no doubt, and not just because of the cardiovascular benefits or the exercise that bicycling provides to the lower limbs. *What an ingenious way to keep the humors moving*, he would have thought.

At the same time, Mercuriale would not have been dismayed if few people here exercised strenuously, regularly, publicly. Just because one *can* does not mean one *should*, he felt very strongly—on the face of it, a puzzling contradiction. In a chapter of his book devoted precisely to this topic, he says of those who think that everyone should exercise, "They are very clearly hallucinating!" Some people are "considerably harmed by physical exercise," he states—the weak, the ill, the "feeble," the elderly among them. Others are not "suited" for it, such as those who are naturally of "hot and moist" temperament. Working up a sweat could throw such people off their humoral balance. Another category went unmentioned: those who would likely never exercise because it would seem beneath their station to do so. During the Renaissance, exercise was identified less closely with health than with labor, manual labor—a turnoff for the nobility, the landed gentry, and the merchant class. (Ironically, these would be the very people most capable of buying Mercuriale's book.)

Unlike in Mercuriale's time, virtually all people nowadays know the benefits of actual, sweat-inducing exercise. Everyone knows. One can hardly be "against" it, really; its overall benefits to physical and mental health are too well documented and widely known by this point. One can *try* to make a case, as the writer Mark Greif did in his 2004 essay "Against Exercise," or as the philosopher Jennifer Michael Hecht did in her 2007 book *The Happiness Myth*. Greif's case, more tongue in cheek than it may have seemed on first reading, is aimed particularly at the modern gym, with its mirrors and gleaming machines, which he likens to "a well-ordered masturbatorium." But he is equally pitiless (and funny) in describing people who exercise in public—runners, for example: "With his speed and narcissistic intensity the runner corrupts the space of walking, thinking, talking, and everyday contacts. He jostles the idler out of his reverie. He races between pedestrians in conversation. The runner can oppose sociability and solitude by publicly sweating on them."

Hecht takes a less pompous and personal (or, personalized) approach—more scientific and historical—marshaling evidence to prove that exercising is not what it's cracked up to be. "In truth," she asserts, "in the context of most of human history, our idea that a good life includes a lot of physical exercise is bizarre." She goes on to observe the myriad contradictions and mixed messages of a culture that would invent both escalators and StairMaster machines, elevators and step classes. What's more, "We expect our coworker to be clean when they get to work, and still clean at the end of the day; yet we also expect them to have a separate wardrobe for the gym, which they drench with sweat. What curious behavior."

Curious, indeed, but to my mind, both commentators give the sense of trying too hard in coming out against exercise—whether to be provocative, clever, cheeky, or simply contrary. This is not to say that exercise is the cure-all that some might say, or that all forms of exercise are healthy, or that too much exercise is always a good thing. In fact, one of the main reasons that people exercise—to lose weight—has also been shown to be one of the least beneficial. One is far more likely to lose weight by drastically reducing calories than by burning them. Twenty minutes on a treadmill at the gym will only burn about three hundred calories—roughly equivalent to one cup of ice cream.

On the other hand, one can dislike exercise, despise it, tire of it, decide never to do it, for a million reasons, while not denying that it is, at least in some respects, good for you. When I first met Silvia Ferretto, the young medical historian who would guide me through Mercuriale's Padua, she seemed uninterested when I told her about my research topic, even dismissive. As for herself, she would rather smoke than exercise, she said, and lit up a Gauloise.

NOT ON A bike but on two feet, and with several stops for cigarette breaks, Dr. Ferretto showed me all of central Padua. Together with a translator named Alberto whom I had hired (Dr. Ferretto spoke no English), we walked the same cobblestone streets that Mercuriale walked when he lived here nearly five hundred years ago. The city was so charming that one could easily understand how Mercuriale must have loved it. Even so, a question remained: Why would he have left behind everything he had achieved in Rome? The life he led there sounded glamorous. He inhabited a palace staffed by attendants and served as private physician to one of the most powerful, wealthy, and, by most accounts, well-liked figures of his time. Mercuriale got to travel by carriage to sumptuous Farnese family vacation homes outside the city and, whether on curial or family business, to destinations throughout Italy. He had access to the world's greatest libraries and, as a sign of the esteem in which he was held, was even named a Citizen of Rome, an honor akin to being given the key to a city.

Glamorous, perhaps, but only in retrospect: Mercuriale was thirty-nine at the time he left Rome and still unmarried, as he had to be in order to live at the Cancelleria, the cardinal's official residence, from which women were barred and where the men were expected to be celibate. Perhaps he simply wished to settle down. (And sure enough, he did: Two years later, in 1571, Mercuriale married Francesca di Bartolomeo Bici, with whom he would have two sons and three daughters.) Perhaps he wished to teach—to bring to the classroom the wisdom of the ancients and the knowledge he'd gained from his wide-ranging reading in researching the *Gymnastica*. And perhaps, too, the sometimes-treacherous waters of the Roman curia got to him, and he was wise to get out before being forced out, like Ligorio, banished to Ferrara. As the historian Richard Palmer has pointed out: "The competition of courtiers for favor encouraged flattery, envy, calumny, rancor, and quarrels, and ultimately led to disappointed hopes." One could feel used like a pawn by those in power, too. In one of the few surviving letters from his years in Rome, Mercuriale insinuates that his boss, Cardinal Farnese, exploited his medical expertise by offering it as a form of patronage—perhaps even as payback, say, for favors done—to anyone he desired.

One thing seems clear: The publication of *De arte gymnastica* was well received and must have played a part in the handsome job offer he received from the University of Padua. He left Rome in the summer of 1569, and on October 6 of that year he officially began what would be an eighteen-year term as the chair of practical medicine. A month later, he held his first class.

Records show that Mercuriale's contract with the university was renewed six years later, and he was given a raise—from six hundred to nine hundred florins annually. Shortly after this, however, a calamity occurred that nearly destroyed his reputation. In August 1575, there was an outbreak of bubonic plague in Venice, less than twenty-five miles away, and Mercuriale was summoned to advise on how to contain it. This did not go well. Mercuriale unwisely counseled against quarantining those who were ill, apparently thinking this would incite more fear. Alas, the epidemic quickly escalated: 50,000 Venetians died (out of a population of 180,000) and about 13,000 Paduans. Mercuriale and other officials were blamed, though not criminally charged, for the terrible toll. To his credit, Mercuriale came to recognize his mistake and wrote about it as a sort of cautionary tale in a subsequent book about dealing with plague, *On Pestilence*— one that we might find relevant today.

ON OUR WALKING tour, we visited the University of Padua and stopped at the famous anatomy theater, restored to its sixteenth-century design; saw a five-hundred-year-old lectern of the sort that Mercuriale would have used in the classroom; and toured the Orto Botanico, the world's oldest academic botanical garden, which Mercuriale used for growing medicinal herbs and in teaching *Materia medica* to his students. But what made the most vivid impression on me was our visit to the University of Padua library. The building itself was nothing special; the administrative office called to mind a Department of Motor Vehicles. But there was an air of history that was unmistakable. The library, having not quite entered the twenty-first century, still used a card catalog, which I loved flipping through—a tactile sensation unlike any other, the card stock thicker than the pages of a book. Under M, I found two dozen cards for Mercuriale volumes and chose three: the first edition of the *Gymnastica*; an eighteenth-century edition; and Mercuriale's book on pediatrics, none of which I had ever seen. Dr. Ferretto conducted some on-the-spot diplomacy to gain permission to see these rare volumes (normally, this would take a week). The librarian scowled and objected—he had to, of course, he couldn't make breaking the rules seem easily permissible—and then just as predictably relented. It would take half an hour to retrieve.

In the meantime, Silvia, Alberto, and I climbed up to the narrow, book-lined catwalk that wrapped around the room's perimeter. Here, in a dusty student registry going back to the sixteenth century, I found records of students whom Mercuriale had tutored while he was chair of practical medicine, a position that came with some unwelcome administrative duties. He had to serve as "protector" (essentially, an advocate) of those who were members of the Natio Germanica Artistarum—an association of students from many parts of northern Europe who came to Padua to study. At one point, his vaunted diplomatic skills were put to the test, however, when the bishop of Padua decreed that these students, primarily Protestant, must participate in Catholic observances, and they angrily protested. Claiming discrimination, they apparently denounced Mercuriale, boycotted his classes, and appealed to Venetian authorities for help. I imagine that he'd had little choice but to abide by the bishop's rules, especially given the severe sectarian atmosphere. But a resolution of some sort was eventually achieved, which must have come as a great relief to Mercuriale. He was not one to risk his own reputation, particularly since sales of his books to students and doctors outside Italy would depend, in part, on his good name.

A desk bell signaled that the requested books had arrived, special passengers on a library version of a dumbwaiter, and we quickly descended to the main floor. Without thinking, I started to reach for the stack of books but found myself body-blocked by a librarian who sharply said something in Italian. Alberto whispered the translation in my ear: "If you drop them, you will have to be beheaded."

I begged his pardon and backed away. The librarian placed the books on a broad desk, and the three of us gathered around. Now, for once, I could be a translator. Neither Silvia nor Alberto had ever heard of Girolamo Mercuriale before that morning.

All three volumes were in flawless condition. How remarkable it was to see a first edition of the 1569 *Gymnastica*: a small book, with its dedication to Cardinal Farnese and its single illustration—the over-sized woodcut of the Vitruvian architectural plan for a gymnasium—folded up carefully inside. Although the exact print run is not known, Dr. Nutton had made a best guess that just five hundred to one thousand copies of this first edition were published.

While I examined the *Gymnastica*, Dr. Ferretto carefully paged through the eighteenth-century edition, published in Amsterdam. It was a much larger book, perhaps a foot and a half by two feet, with beautiful heavy paper and lavish illustrations—more elaborate versions of the illustrations Ligorio had done. Everything looked a little overdone, rococo in style, as identifiably eighteenth century as the austere 1569 edition was of the late Renaissance.

Whispering, Dr. Ferretto read aloud several of the chapter titles from the *Gymnastica*, translating from the Latin: "When to Exercise," "How Much Exercise Should One Get," "On the Nature of Running," "A Refutation of Those Who Think Everyone Should Exercise." She shook her head as if not quite believing this was real—*really* from five hundred years before. Was it possible that Dr. Mercuriale just might convert her to try some exercise? Watching as someone else, someone other than me, responded to this book was deeply satisfying.

We said goodbyes and parted ways after the library, and I found a bar near Piazza Signori to get a slice of pizza. As I waited and sipped a beer, a young Italian man made his order to the bartender. He emptied all the change from his pockets and, not coming up with enough, dug out a euro note tucked beneath an ID card in his wallet—as if this were literally his last dollar.

Clearly a student, I thought to myself. Soon, a throng of other students joined the young man, fifteen or twenty, their avid faces calling to mind those students who were so devoted to Mercuriale that they would take down every word of his lectures and turn them into books like *De decoratione liber*. Within ten minutes, however, the students were gone: the bar emptied as they went outside for a smoke—not just one or two lone smokers consigned to the sidewalk, as in America, but all of them, puffing away happily, laughing, debating. It looked so convivial I almost wanted to join them.

The Rest Principle

As for athletic training, we assert that it is a form of wisdom.

—PHILOSTRATUS, CA. A.D. 220

Another crowd of students, another street scene. Not burnished, parti-colored Padua this time, but midtown Manhattan, on a rainy, cold morning in late October 2011. And in place of Italian undergraduates, twenty-five suspiciously fit young men and women—and me—just waiting. No one is smoking.

That this particular building would be closed on a Saturday was to be expected: it was a gym that was only open during the work week. That the door was locked, however, and that no one could be reached to open it suggested that there had been a screw-up. Our instructor, a wholesome-looking fellow in a trench coat, confirmed this to the small crowd. He fumed silently but expressively—eyes flaring, jaw clenched—bringing to mind a parish priest who'd been locked out of his own church.

Finally, some twenty minutes later a gym employee appeared and, apologizing for oversleeping, unlocked the door and let us in. Coats were hung, umbrellas left to dry, and we filed into an aerobics studio still redolent of last night's sweat. Folding chairs and a projection screen had been set up. When the lights were turned off, I had a sense of déjà vu as the first slide flashed on-screen: "HUMAN ANATOMY: The Science Dealing with the Structure of the Human Body." In what seemed like a lifetime ago, I had attended a yearlong course on human anatomy as research for my book *The Anatomist*. It had been held in an enormous lecture hall at a major university in San Francisco, where the students were studying to be doctors. Those of us gathered in an otherwise empty New York gym were in pursuit of a tangentially related but less eminent profession: to become certified personal fitness trainers.

I did not plan to train people professionally but hoped to learn what one must learn to *become* a trainer, and to build on my layman's knowledge of exercise, anatomy, and kinesiology. Others were definitely there to start a new career. They were dancers, actors, ex-jocks (male and female alike), and waitresses and bartenders who no longer wanted to wait tables and tend bar. Over the next eight weeks, we would attend classes from nine A.M. to five P.M. every Saturday and Sunday—over 120 hours of study.

Our instructor introduced himself and began his lecture. What we first saw on-screen was not all that different from what one would have seen illustrated some four hundred years earlier in Vesalius's *Fabrica*: a literal muscle man, a body stripped of skin to show the topmost layer of muscles beneath. Memorizing the main muscles of the human body and, more to the point, understanding their role, location, and function would be a foundation of our learning. As important as knowing what muscles help us do—lift, jump, squat, lunge, flex—would be fully appreciating what they *prevent* us from doing: falling apart, folding in on oneself, crashing to the floor. The lumbar spine provides the only skeletal support between the rib cage and the hips, for instance, so most other support for this area comes from the muscles that make up the abdominal wall. Running three layers deep in front and on each side, the abs help contain major organs of the digestive system—like the top of a Tupperware container sealed tight—and help one stand upright.

Muscles get the lion's share of credit and attention when it comes to exercise, but the reality is that movement—exercise at its essence—actually occurs at joints. These come in six types: ball-and-socket, hinge, condyloid, pivot, gliding, and saddle joints. The movements they make can be defined by the plane in space along, or within, which they take place: the frontal plane (side to side movements), sagittal (flexion and extension), and transverse (twisting and rotating). These planes are not seen, obviously—they have to be envisioned—but once one is aware of them, one sees the body, movement, and working out differently. Ideally, a workout is based on different planes of movement, not merely on different body parts. So, on a "chest day," you wouldn't want to perform only exercises in the transverse plane—presses, push-ups, and so on. Instead, you want to mix in exercises that involve other planes of movement, other directions, creating a dynamism that will help shape your body more symmetrically and will, incidentally, be kinder to your joints.

Whereas in the anatomy lab my classmates and I dissected human bodies, our practical task on that first day of class was to dissect human movement. Enough with the slides and questions; the instructor had us break into small groups and assigned a specific exercise for each to analyze anatomically—lunge, bench press, pull-up, biceps curl, and so on—after which we would report back to class. Some went into the gym to analyze the movements involved in weightlifting, cycling, and running. My group got what one might consider a deceptively simple exercise: the mechanics of a standing squat.

MY CLASSMATES AND I left the gym at the end of our first day with a greater appreciation of the complexity of movement, not to mention a lot of reading to do before returning the next morning. We had two textbooks: a 550-page manual on strength and fitness training, and a workbook customized for the course. One might think such texts are a recent phenomenon, like the field of exercise science itself, but this is not so. Two millennia ago, the prominent Greek teacher and philosopher Flavius Philostratus wrote what is considered the first book on physical fitness training. Its title: *Gymnasticus* (or, *On Gymnastics*).

The book is unlike Mercuriale's for a number of reasons. Philostratus was not a physician, and hence his book was not a medical text. Also, his focus was on training for athletes, not on the pros and cons of various forms of exercise that may be used prescriptively for any person.

The text was likely written between A.D. 220 and 230, when the author was a man of about fifty. (He would live to around age eighty.) This was well past the golden age of the Hellenic Empire; Greece was now under Roman rule. While athletic festivals and games, like the Olympics, continued, and the culture of gymnasia and baths continued in Rome as in Athens, a shift in attitude was underway; relatively speaking, it would not be long before the culture of athletics would disappear, as Christianity became a predominant force. This is a key to understanding the text, which is partly a defense of the ancient Greek art of athletic training.

But it is more than that—or, shall I say, more pointed. Philostratus's text is also a stinging rebuke to Galen, the physician whose work dates from just before this period (Galen died ca. A.D. 210). In his writing, Galen is scathing in his critique of athletic trainers, of which two distinct types were recognized at the time: the *paidotribe* (equivalent to a personal fitness or athletic trainer) and the *gymnaste* (a specialist providing advice on exercise, diet, and massage). In his translation for the recent Loeb Classical Library edition of Philostratus's text, the scholar Jason König explains that "for Galen . . . the trainers are an extreme example of the way in which medical incompetence can masquerade as expertise." He was defending his turf against quacks, as he felt that trainers threatened "to encroach on his medical expertise by claiming medical skills they do not possess and in the process do enormous damage to the bodies of their charges." In articulating this view, Galen aligned himself with Hippocrates and Plato. Philostratus begged to differ.

Trivial as it might seem to some today, Philostratus's argument was no small thing. Defending the views or work of trainers meant disagreeing with, if not contradicting, the words of the fathers of medicine and philosophy. But Philostratus seems to have been fearless in entering such a debate. Exactly why he would do so is not entirely clear. He wasn't himself a trainer, nor does he speak of his own history of athletics or exercise. It was more about upholding honor, tradition, while also seizing on a topic that he could sink his teeth into.

"I have decided to . . . contribute for trainers and their subjects alike everything I know, and to defend nature, which is critical because the athletes of today are inferior to those of former times." He goes on to explain that it's not athletes who have changed but athletic training: "It is the lack of healthy training and vigorous exercise that have deprived nature of her strength."

In the book's opening passage, Philostratus pulls no punches, invoking the words of Galen and Plato for his own purposes: "As for athletic training, we assert that it is a form of wisdom, and one that is inferior to none of the other skills [such as poetry and music], which means it can be summed up in treatise form for the benefit of those who wish to undertake training."

But he also sides with Galen when it comes to serious medical problems being the province of specially trained physicians: "If someone has a break or a flesh wound or clouding of the sight in his eyes or a dislocation of one of his limbs, then he needs to be taken to the doctor, for the art of the athletic trainer does not concern itself with problems of those kinds."

Within the text, which runs to about ten thousand words, Philostratus pauses to consider the kind of man who makes an excellent trainer—and for him only a man will do, by the way. To make this point, Philostratus tells a story, possibly apocryphal, of a woman from Rhodes who trained her son in boxing for athletic competition at Olympia, a deception that was not allowed. Apparently, she looked and acted so much like a man, as Philostratus put it, that no one knew she was his mother. After she was found out, "a law was written that the trainer must strip naked" to prove that he was male when working with an athlete at Olympia.

Philostratus goes on: "Let us have a look now at the trainer himself, to see what sort of man will supervise the athlete, and what the extent of his knowledge will be. Let the trainer be neither garrulous nor untrained in speech," so that he can properly motivate his athletes. The trainer also needs to know his charges well, "being a sort of judge of the athlete's nature. Indeed he should know all the signs of character in the eyes, by which are revealed lazy people." Philostratus emphasized that trainers must know "the whole art of physiognomy . . . The characteristics of the parts of the body are also to be considered, as in the art of sculpture."

While Philostratus states that his text is intended to preserve knowledge of the ancient art of training, one learns more about what not to do as a trainer than what to do. His text does not contain specific exercise regimens or programs, for instance. However, it does include more than one cautionary tale about training taken too far. In one case, this resulted in a trainer killing his athlete with a "sharpened strigil as a punishment for not exercising endurance in the pursuit of victory." In another anecdote—again, possibly apocryphal—Philostratus says that a trainer killed an athlete through overexertion: "The trainer became angry and listened furiously and was irritable with him on the grounds that he was relaxing his training and interrupting the tetrads [a system of training according to a rigid, preplanned four-day cycle], until he actually killed the athlete through his training, out of ignorance, by not prescribing the exercises he should have chosen even if the athlete had said nothing about his condition."

THE EIGHT-WEEK COURSE in personal training went by in a blur. Since I was working full-time at a day job, my nights were filled with studying biomechanics, basic physiology, kinesiology, and more. Indeed, this was a time in my life when I more often took flash cards than lovers to bed. And when I did take lovers, I dissected them with my eyes and quizzed them: Is this your femur or your tibia? May I please palpate your gluteus medius? I always pointed out the beauty of the inguinal canals, the twin lines right below the waist where the lower abdominals meet the pubic area.

My career didn't depend on my passing the final exam, but my self-respect did. The oldest guy in the class couldn't be the only one who failed. Fortunately, I passed with a respectable score and received my certification. All these years later, I still recall the six principles on which a long-term personal fitness training program can be built—a major part of our final exam. Not because I have a stellar memory, but because, in each of these concepts I found a correlative to my work, my passion—to writing—although they could apply equally well to just about any vocation or endeavor.

First, there is the Principle of Specificity. This states that what you train for is what you get: If it is strength you want, train for strength. In short, be specific in your work goals as much as in your workouts. It's all in the details.

Next, the Overload Principle: train a part of the body above the level to which it is accustomed. You must provide constant stimuli, so the body never gets used to a given task; otherwise, expect no change. Push yourself, in other words, try new things, whether at the gym, at your desk, or in the office—creative cross-training, one might say.

This leads to the Principle of Progression. Once you master new tasks, move on. Don't get stuck—whether on a given task or an exercise regimen. If you do, this will lead to the Principle of Accommodation. With no new demands placed on it, the body accommodates or reaches homeostasis—not a good place to find oneself. So don't get too comfortable; it will show in your work as clearly as in the mirror.

When stimuli are removed, gains are reversed—use it or lose it, as the Principle of Reversibility emphasizes. Just as movement in any form is better than none at all—walk around the block if you can't make it to spin class—one must do something, anything, to keep the creative and intellectual motors running.

And finally, the Rest Principle, the tenet that gave me particular solace. To make fitness gains, whether in strength, speed, stamina, or whatever your aim (see Principle of Specificity), you must take ample time to recover.

I had been working out as long as I had been writing, so this last principle was not new to me. But I had never observed this rule very strictly when it came to working on a piece of writing. Just as the body needs time to rest, so does an essay, story, chapter, poem, or especially, a book.

In some cases, it's not just the writing that needs a breather but the writer, too. After completing my book *The Anatomist*, I wrote virtually nothing for almost three years. I hadn't given up writing deliberately, and I cannot pinpoint a particular day when my not-writing period started, any more than one can say the moment when one is overtaken by sleep. It's only after you wake that you realize how long you were out.

Nor did I feel "blocked" at first. Lines would come to me and then slip away, like a dog that loses interest in how you are petting it and seeks another hand. This goes both ways. When I lost interest in them, the lines gradually stopped coming.

I didn't miss writing, yet I felt something missing—a phantom voice, one might say. I had been pursuing writing since I was a teenager, had published pieces in many places, and had written three books back-to-back. To have silence and neither deadlines nor expectations for the first time in years was sort of nice—and sort of troubling. Can one call oneself a writer when not-writing is what one actually does, day after day?

I never lied. If someone asked, I would say that I wasn't working on anything and no, had nothing on the back burner, in the oven, cooking, percolating, or marinating. (What's with all the food metaphors anyway?) I wasn't hungry either. But I was tired. Very tired. And thinking about the "Rest Principle" helped me find my way back to writing and provided validation for what I had done instinctively. On this matter, I quote from the National Council on Strength and Fitness training manual, one of the textbooks we used in our course: "As the rate of motor unit fatigue increases, the effect becomes more pronounced, causing performance to decline proportionately to the level of fatigue . . . During the recovery period, the muscle fibers can rebuild their energy reserves, fix any damage resulting from the production of force, and fully return to normal pre-exertion levels."

Translation: Don't work through the pain; it will only hurt. Give yourself sufficient time to refresh.

How long should this period be? What is true for muscle fibers is true for creative ones as well. My rule of thumb in fitness training is two-to-one: for every two days of intense workouts, a day off. However, "in cases of sustained high-level output," according to my manual, full recovery may take longer. This is what had happened with me creatively. I needed a really, really long rest.

Then one day a line came to me. It didn't slip away this time but stayed put. I followed it, like a path. It led to another, then another.

Soon, pieces started lining up in my head, like cabs idling curb-side, ready to go where I wanted to take them. But it wasn't so much that pages started getting written that made me realize my not-writing period had come to an end. Instead, my perspective had shifted. Writing is not measured in page counts, any more than a writer is defined by publication credits. To succeed at any endeavor, whatever it may be, is to make a commitment to the long haul, as one does to keeping fit and healthy for as long as possible. For me, this meant staying active both physically and creatively, switching it up, remaining curious and interested in learning new skills—I took up photography—and of course giving myself ample periods of rest. I knew that the writer in me, like the fitness devotee, would be better off.

Esercizio a Roma

Many points have escaped this learned doctor;
it would be better if he had never written anything.

—Joseph Scaliger, Dutch historian,
on Girolamo Mercuriale, ca. 1604

Although visiting Milan and Padua had been a quick, spontaneous trip, just a few months later I was able to return to Italy for five weeks as a visiting scholar at the American Academy in Rome. My goal: to follow in Mercuriale's footsteps, to get a feel for the place where he lived and worked and wrote *De arte gymnastica*. The academy not only provided wonderful accommodations but also the resources of the institution itself—the library, the staff, the fellow scholars and artists, many of whom were fluent in Italian and would be able to help me navigate the city. I had been eager to get inside the Palazzo della Cancelleria, where Mercuriale actually lived, but I found that it remains a Papal Chancellery and is not accessible to outsiders, scholars and tourists alike. The Palazzo Farnese, on the other hand, now houses the French Embassy and provides guided tours of the interior. I set out to investigate on one of my first days in Rome.

It was a short walk down the hill and across the Tiber. The Palazzo, closed on weekends and guarded by fierce-looking armed soldiers, dominated a small piazza near the Campo de' Fiori. I found it to be a huge, imposing block of a building, neither beautiful nor ugly, and not in the least ornate. Indeed, there was something inscrutable about it in its orderliness and architectural restraint. But the Palazzo Farnese, built in the early sixteenth century, was no less a palace for not being ostentatious. What came to mind was a vault, an enormous bank vault: behind those solid walls, there must have been incredible stores of wealth and history and power.

Back at the academy, an architectural historian who knew Rome and its buildings well sketched out for me the three-story palazzo's basic floor plans and made a guess as to where the legendary Farnese library might have been located: most likely on an upper floor rather than in the basement, where hundreds of servants and other workers probably lived.

That night, during the old-fashioned cocktail hour that precedes dinner in the formal dining room—a time to mingle and socialize over a Negroni—I literally bumped into Alice Waters, the legendary founding chef of Berkeley's Chez Panisse. She was in residence for a few weeks as part of her long-standing involvement with the Rome Sustainable Food Project (founded under her guidance in 2007), which utilized the academy's own extensive vegetable garden and advocated on behalf of local farmers and organic suppliers for other institutions and restaurants in Rome. We had met a few times before, years earlier, when I lived in the Bay Area. After I told her what I was working on here in Rome, Alice looked puzzled, bothered even. She had thought exercise was purely a modern construct, and she didn't look at all happy to hear me explain that gyms actually existed thousands of years ago, including here in Rome. To her mind, gyms were terrible places: "Gyms are the fast food of exercise," she declared. How unpleasant it is, she observed, that people think they must go to a gym to exercise: "Nothing comes of it, nothing is produced as a result. People have lost the association between exercise and manual work, exercise and nature!" Alice's instantaneous passion on the topic was as unexpected as it was invigorating.

"Every morning, I wake up at seven o'clock and I go out the door and I walk for forty-five minutes," she went on to say. "Wherever I am, however I am feeling. I don't see what the weather is like, I just walk. And it gives me time to think through my day, and then I return and I get organized for work. I always, always learn something."

She added that she would love to see what she has done with food—at her Berkeley restaurant, in Rome, and beyond—translated into a philosophy of exercise: incorporated into one's day, naturally, pleasurably, without effort, without artifice, without extravagance, without—she did not use this word, and I hesitated to tell her the title of my book—*sweat*. "It's the difference between going to a gym and dancing: one is work, the other is pleasurable." Perhaps it is this word, *exercise*, that is so daunting, Alice noted: "In my life, it has always been part of my work: carrying boxes up from the basement to the restaurant, sweeping the steps, going up and down the stairs: not thinking about it as this other thing, this separate thing—a place one has to go."

I thought about how exercise supposedly "disappeared" during the Middle Ages, and how this was not exactly true. Exercise did not go extinct or die; it was simply not separated out, promoted so self-consciously, as it was during antiquity and is today. Except for the wealthy, people did sweep their floors, carry their goods and produce, work in the garden—move, from the time they woke until they rested. And they danced. As Mercuriale himself points out in a chapter titled "The Purpose and Place of Dancing," human beings have always danced, if not for exercise per se, then for its social aspects and for the pure pleasure to be found in rhythmically moving one's body. A near-contemporary of Mercuriale's, the Venetian physiologist and physician known as Santorio Santorio, agreed, albeit with a note of caution: "Moderate dancing without Jumping, comes the nearest of anything to the Advantages of Walking," he observed in his book of aphorisms, "for it leisurely expels the digested perspirable Matter."

Alice made a connection to the philosophy of another Italian physician and teacher, Maria Montessori. (Before Chez Panisse, Alice taught at a Montessori school.) "In Montessori, they teach that there is 'work' and there is 'play,' and both are important. But the way it is now, exercise is in this category of 'work' and that's not where it should be—as if one has to work for good health. No. Good health shouldn't be the goal of exercise. Make 'pleasure' the goal"—as in dancing—"and it will lead to good health."

I was intrigued and stimulated by Alice's views: giving up the gym, slowing down, not speeding up, going outside, getting the body moving, whatever the weather, not staying in, and dancing more; a slow burn, not a competitive one. It seemed to me the epitome of "going local," local being your own body—viewing one's body as the ultimate sustainable resource.

A FEW DAYS later, I returned to the Palazzo Farnese, planning only to make an appointment to visit the library—standard protocol, as I had been advised by one of the academy's librarians, who had provided the letter of introduction required for entrance. When I reached the building's grand front door, however, the armed guards paid me no mind whatsoever. Three men had arrived at the exact same time, and one guy punched a code into the door keypad. The gigantic door slowly opened—softly, widely, like lips welcoming a kiss. I slipped in with them, and the door closed, just as softly, behind me. Following the three men's lead, I went through security and then waited in line at the reception desk. Holding my letter of introduction from the academy in front of me like a hired driver at an airport holding a sign, I inquired about making an appointment. The man behind the counter replied casually, "Si, piano due," and pointed to a massive stone stairway to the second floor. There, a librarian glanced at my letter, gave me a map and a password for Wi-Fi (*wee-fee*, as she pronounced it), and—"Allora!"—to my surprise, welcomed me in.

Within minutes, I found myself sitting at a desk in Sale 3, Piano 2, of the library in Palazzo Farnese, facing a window that looked out onto the open courtyard and the sky. I was one of hundreds of people there, primarily students of the French school housed in this building.

Books surrounded me. Granted, these were not the same books that Mercuriale had access to, not the exact same Farnese library, but the atmosphere must have been, to some degree, comparable. There was total silence but for footsteps—the sound of footsteps on the stone floors; otherwise, I heard no talking, no whispering. It struck me that there are different kinds of silence: some libraries impose a tense, brittle silence, a pompous silence, a silence enforced by security guards and rules. By contrast, this was a silence of studying, of students, a silence of readers, of reading. I imagined that this was the kind of silence Mercuriale enjoyed while researching and writing the *Gymnastica* in that very building.

I moved to another room, if only because I could. I decided I was going to sit in every room that Mercuriale himself might have sat in.

I was now on the west side, with the sky to my right. On my left: shelf after shelf after shelf of books, books to the ceiling, the highest shelves reached by a catwalk surrounding the room, made accessible by delicate spiral staircases in the corners.

I took a staircase up to the catwalk and picked a volume off a shelf at random: *Past and Present: A Journal of Historical Studies*. I opened it and happened upon a review of the contemporary multivolume French work, *A History of the Body*.

Huh.

The title got me thinking about my own work. A history of exercise is not really—or certainly not only—a history of the body. It is, equally, perhaps even primarily, a history of the *mind*—of will, desire, self-discipline—for one cannot get exercise without an intentional wish, a motivation, a reason, to do so. As Mercuriale himself argued, it is the *intention* that makes an activity exercise, rather than simply work. With that, I dropped to the ground beneath me, right there on the library catwalk, and did as many push-ups as rapidly and silently as I could.

THE BEAUTY OF a push-up is that it involves virtually the entire body, requires no machinery other than the human body, tones muscle, and, if done energetically, has a cardiovascular effect. To begin, you assume the plank position—arms extended with elbows locked, shoulders over wrists, back straight, legs fully extended, toes tucked under, and head relaxed, eyes to the ground. Maintaining stability, preventing the body from collapsing or curling in on itself, is a feat in itself. This demands active engagement of the muscles of the back (rhomboids and trapezius—between the shoulder blades), trunk (all the abdominal muscles, plus the stabilizing muscles of the spine), neck, and shoulders. If you did nothing more than this—just holding this plank position for as long as you could, whether thirty seconds or three minutes—you would be doing your body a favor, performing an isometric exercise.

To lower the prone body to the floor and push back up involves the two muscles of the biceps, the three in the triceps group, and those of the forearm. The chest muscles (pectoralis major and minor) are crucial as well for maintaining stability. The ball-and-socket joint at the shoulder rotates, thus placing a push-up in the transverse plane.

Through this anatomical lens, one has a better appreciation for why a push-up is generally more challenging for a woman than a man. It calls especially on the muscles of the upper body, which are usually less developed or prominent in women. Even so, a woman can do a push-up as well as a man, though this may require taking it in stages. I once had the privilege to meet the late Supreme Court justice Ruth Bader Ginsburg, eighty-one at the time, and when I took the opportunity to ask about her personal exercise regime, she gave me a surprising response.

"Every day, I do twenty push-ups," she told me.

This was notable for several reasons: First, to do push-ups every day is a demonstration of discipline that few can claim. Second, twenty is a good number for anyone—but particularly for a person who is eighty-one. "That is remarkable," I told her.

The Supreme Court justice shrugged it off. "At first I couldn't do any," she said, "not a single one." She started by doing them standing against a wall. Next, she moved to push-ups poised on the knees, and finally to a full military push-up. This wasn't of her own initiative, she hastened to add. She had worked out with a personal trainer since her treatment for cancer in 1999.

"He saved my life," Justice Ginsburg said matter-of-factly. At the time we spoke, she was working out with him twice a week. I pictured private sessions at home, but she clarified that she would go to a small gym housed in the Supreme Court building—always at the end of the workday, seven to eight P.M., roughly. She would warm up on an elliptical machine while watching the news, then her trainer would take her through a workout including dumbbells, stretch cords, weight machines, and body-weight exercises such as push-ups and standing squats.

"When I was on the Court of Appeals, I used to go to a Jazzercise class," she added. The very thought of the Notorious RBG doing Jazzercise made me admire her even more. I could easily imagine this petite, fine-boned woman moving elegantly, lithely. But the Jazzercise music was not to her taste—she was an opera buff—and she eventually stopped going.

She spoke of all this with no embarrassment or self-consciousness, and, indeed, I felt somehow she enjoyed talking about exercise, at least for a short time. When I said goodnight and thanked her, I added, "I'm going to go home and do twenty push-ups."

"You're young and healthy," Justice Ginsburg said in her throaty whisper. "You can do a lot more than that."

A Physical Education

*Exercise is so much more helpful and invigorating when
the mind is interested, than when it is not.*

—CATHARINE BEECHER, *A TREATISE ON DOMESTIC
ECONOMY*, 1848

A week before I was scheduled to leave Rome, I decided to fly to
Stockholm for two days. I had discovered that one of the most
influential figures in the history of exercise, Pehr Henrik Ling, had
lived and worked in Stockholm during the early nineteenth century;
that the training institute Ling founded in 1813 still exists in the same
location, now as a college for exercise science; and that Stockholm is
home to major collections of rare books on exercise, sports, and
physical culture. Although Ling is hardly a household name, he is
better known than a figure like Mercuriale because his philosophy of
exercise had a direct impact on shifts in attitude toward exercise in
the nineteenth century, particularly when it came to women and to
PE instruction for children, not only in Sweden but around the

world. Ling and his many disciples were complex figures, and I was determined to learn more about them.

ON MY FLIGHT to Stockholm, there was a baby boy in his mother's arms in the seat in front of mine. His face bobbed above the headrest, comically, as she bounced him up and down to quiet him. He was maybe four months old. I waved at him and smiled. He responded, reached through the crack between seats, and grabbed for my finger. I let him. His grip was strong—*strong*! Four tiny fingers around my meaty index finger. He let go and gripped again, let go and gripped again. His brain and neuromuscular system were learning. He was practicing this move—exercising, in a sense. This is how it begins, I thought to myself. I could see how he enjoyed it—the gripping, the exertion put on the muscles in his fingers and hand, the satisfaction of letting go, the interaction with a fellow human. He giggled, and a whole range of emotions animated his pudgy face as he went through this cycle of movements. He poked his little arm through over and over and over again to squeeze my finger.

I arrived in Stockholm in the late afternoon. It was very cold, yet the air was as dry as in a sauna, unlike the wet, slushy winters in New York. There was no snow on the ground; it was just bitterly cold—and dark. I bundled up and headed out after I checked into my hotel. A Swedish friend had recommended a favorite restaurant, a bus ride and a short walk away. The spotless streets were nearly empty, so unlike Rome. I had trouble finding anyone at all to point me in the right direction when I lost my way. But at last I did reach my destination, a tiny restaurant called Sardin, and took a seat at the jammed bar. I ordered a beer, and the bartender and I got to talking. I explained why I'd come to Stockholm, and she—like so many others on this journey—looked completely stumped. "I can't help you with that," she said at last. She plucked a chocolate from a bowl on the bar, unwrapped it, and popped it in her mouth. "This is what I do. Every day: eat chocolate. I take it very seriously."

Two well-dressed, middle-aged Swedish women sat on bar stools right next to me. They were discreetly chatting for a time, and then a fascinating physiological phenomenon occurred, one that is unique to humans in its multiple manifestations. Both women began laughing at something one had said, the other interjected an apparently irresistible detail more, and suddenly their twinned laughter reached the highest altitude of laughterness, like a roller coaster shooting to the top of a loop and then plunging off the rails. Their bodies were virtually taken hostage by laughter: tears streamed down their ruddy cheeks; they were unable to talk, hardly able to breathe, heaving and rocking on their stools, they were laughing so hard. It was as contagious as a yawn. I started laughing, too, although I hadn't understood a word either had said. Finally, one caught her breath while the other was still at the tail end of her giggles: "It's liberating to laugh!" she exclaimed to me in English as she wiped tears with a napkin. "Oh yes, it's always good to laugh," her friend added with a hiccup, and I thought to myself, *Yes, always.* Laughing is not only good for your spirits, erasing cares and woes; it is good exercise, too.

What makes you laugh starts in the brain—you see, hear, or maybe even smell, touch, or taste something that strikes you as funny. The "striking" part is key: an element of surprise, of not expecting it, is at play. For although laughing can be expected—let's say you go to see a stand-up comic, or have drinks with a funny friend—it cannot be induced on command. Whatever way something strikes you as humorous, the somatic response is nearly all-encompassing, head to toe. "Similar to aerobic exercise, a hearty laugh involves contraction and relaxation of facial, chest, abdominal and skeletal muscles," reports Lindsay Wilson-Barlow, a psychiatrist with the Neuropsychiatric Institute at the University of Utah who has studied the physiology of laughter. (This scientific discipline even has a name, gelotology, from the Greek root for laughter, *gelos*, which, incidentally, is also the name for the Greek god of laughter, Gelos, and is etymologically related to *gelatin*, which of course jiggles—or is it giggles?)

"Within the first ten seconds of laughter, fifteen facial muscles contract and relax while stimulation of the zygomatic major muscle (the main lifting mechanism of your upper lip) occurs. In extreme cases, the face may become red or purple," Wilson-Barlow adds. This indicates that facial arteries and capillaries are suddenly flushed with fresh blood, almost as if an injury has taken place and repair work must be done immediately. Even the arm, leg, and trunk muscles get involved in laughing, and of course the entire circulatory system. "Studies have shown that simply twenty seconds of laughter has the ability to double heart rate for the following three to five minutes." Norman Cousins—a journalist who conducted a personal investigation into laughter's healing effects in the 1960s—aptly described laughter as "a form of jogging for the innards." I would take it a step further, given how powerfully the abdominal muscles contract, and say that a round of robust laughter is equivalent to (and perhaps as effective as) doing a quick set of sit-ups.

To a certain extent, Mercuriale recognized this overall effect, too. Laughter, he observed in the *Gymnastica*, "agitates our bodies and exercises them considerably. For who has not seen all the innards of people shake when they laugh, the face lights up, and the head and chest shake?" As a physician, he recommended laughter for a range of conditions, some of which make a certain sense (it's good for those suffering melancholy, grief, or sadness) and some of which do not (laughter as medicine for "madness" caused by "cold humors in the brain"). By contrast with laughter, he concluded, "the body derives little or no benefit from crying." Why the double standard here—since crying also involves shaking, tears, muscular contractions, and facial flushing? Mercuriale offered no explanation.

LAUGHTER ANIMATED AND nearly dominated another space, a less likely one, the next morning, my first day at the library of the Swedish School of Sport and Health Science (as it's called in English), the college founded by Pehr Henrik Ling. And not just laughter but chatter at every table, all filled with students. Many were talking on their cellphones or engaged in vigorous conversations. The atmosphere was closer to a cafeteria than any library I'd been in. I wasn't irritated so much as fascinated. I asked the school librarian, Lotta, about the unique atmosphere. She was matter-of-fact in response: "We don't want to be librarians who always say, 'Be quiet!'" This was their library and they could do as they wished, she implied. Furthermore, Lotta noted, "We are very restricted here in Sweden"—a reference, I presumed, to unwritten rules governing social norms—"so we do what we can to undo the rules."

"I like that," I told her, and alongside the other students, I got to work.

I had been able to order about fifty books in advance of my visit. Lotta had them all lined up and ready for me on a cart when I arrived first thing in the morning. She placed a clean white pillow on the tabletop—a soft bed for these often fragile volumes—and provided a fresh package of hand wipes. Lotta asked me to clean my fingers before and after I examined each one.

What I had before me could pass for the greatest hits in the Western history of exercise. It wasn't everything obviously—every single topic, every author who wrote on the subject—but it certainly served as an excellent overview of writings from the early to late modern periods.

For the moment, I skipped over Arcangelo Tuccaro's 1599 book on "tumbling" and dance, *Trois dialogues de l'exercice de sauter et voltiger en l'air*; the German gymnastics instructor Johann Georg Pascha's small book from 1666 on pommel horse vaulting, *Gründliche Beschreibung des Voltiger (Thorough Descriptions of the Vault)*; and the hefty, eighteenth-century tomes by German writers to get my hands on the library's edition of Ling's *Gymnastikens Allmänna Grunder (The Basics of Gymnastics)*, his one and only book on exercise, published in 1840, the year after his death. In some ways, this beat-up volume of around two hundred pages was disappointing. But if it looked far smaller, shorter, shabbier, and more modest than I had expected, perhaps that's because Ling's broader influence as a figurehead looms so large.

FULLY APPRECIATING LING'S contribution requires first taking into account how dramatically ideas about medicine, science, and physics—indeed, about the workings of the human body and one's very sense of self in the universe—had changed since Mercuriale's day. During the period now known as the Scientific Revolution, dating from the early seventeenth to roughly the mid-eighteenth century, a series of discoveries upended utterly mistaken ideas that had held sway since antiquity. One of the first and most important milestones was the English physician William Harvey's *Exercitatio anatomica de motu cordis et sanguinis in animalibus (On the Motion of the Heart and the Blood)* published in 1628. In this seventy-two-page treatise, considered radical at the time, Harvey drew on experiments he had done on both animals and human subjects, and laid out in logical detail the role of the heart in circulating blood throughout the body via the arteries, veins, and lungs. The evidence was undeniable. Harvey's conception of the circulatory system served as a long-overdue corrective to Galenism and the theory of the four humors, by which Mercuriale and all physicians had abided for more than fifteen centuries. Unsurprisingly, it still took many decades before Harvey's theory was fully embraced by the scientific and medical establishment and Galenism was put to rest at last. Even then, it took far longer for age-old and wrong-headed practices related to humoral theory, such as bloodletting, to die out.

Later in the seventeenth century, the Dutch scientist Antonie van Leeuwenhoek crafted some of the earliest powerful microscopes, leading to his surprising discovery of otherwise invisible organisms such as bacteria—microscopic life. Building on the pioneering Dutchman's work, the Italian biologist and microscopist Marcello Malpighi—often called the father of physiology—was the first to identify capillaries and understand the link they provide between arteries and veins. He was also among the first to study red blood cells, which ferry oxygen to every part of the body. Meanwhile, a fellow Italian scientist, Giovanni Borelli, was conducting ground-breaking studies on what we would now call biomechanics, experiments that culminated in his 1680–81 treatise, *De motu animalium* (*On the Movement of Animals*). His work was notable not only for its scientific analysis of how muscles work and limbs move but also for its virtual dissection of different forms of exercise, including running, jumping, and swimming.

The discoveries made by Harvey, Borelli, and numerous others—including, of course, Sir Isaac Newton's formulation of the laws of motion and of universal gravity in 1687—subsequently influenced the intellectual, philosophical, and social movement of the Enlightenment. It was in this milieu that three eighteenth-century German educators—Christian Gotthilf Salzmann, Johann Gutsmuths, and Friedrich Ludwig Jahn—entered the picture. They were profoundly shaped by the scientific mindset of their time, as well as by the era's major theorists of child development. In 1693, John Locke had published *Some Thoughts Concerning Education*, in which, among other things, he had advocated incorporating physical exercise into school curricula.

("A Sound Mind in a Sound Body, is a short, but full Description of a Happy State in this World," Locke observed.) Also important for Salzmann, Gutsmuths, and Jahn was Jean-Jacques Rousseau's *Emile, or On Education*, from 1762, on the role of the individual in society.

Salzmann founded an innovative school in 1784, the Schnepfenthal Educational Institute, where exercise was a key part of the curriculum, as important as learning geography or foreign languages—a notion influenced by the writings of Rousseau. Gutsmuths joined Salzmann's staff two years later, assuming respon- sibility for the physical education program, a position he retained for over fifty years. Through his leadership at the school and, more significant, through pedagogical manuals such as his seven- hundred-page *Gymnastik für die Jugend* (*Gymnastics for Youth*) from 1793, Gutsmuths's message about the importance of physical educa- tion classes began to spread beyond Germany.

A young Danish man who had studied Gutsmuths's method took his teachings to the next level by opening what is considered the first gym of the modern era in 1799. Franz Nachtegall's small gym in Copenhagen reportedly included rope ladders, climbing poles, balance beams, a wooden horse for vaulting, and floor mats. Though he had only 5 young male students when he started out, by 1804 he reportedly had 150. One of these was Ling, who had moved to Copenhagen the same year Nachtegall opened his gym and stayed on for five years, studying both the Danish and German schools of exercise.

Along with advances in science, medicine, physical education, and understanding of the human body, there was a far more urgent concern prompting the revival of physical fitness specifically in northern European countries at this time: I would call it the Napoleon Effect. As Napoleon moved swiftly, ruthlessly, to conquer territories yet outside his empire in the early years of the 1800s, countries at risk of invasion, such as Sweden, Denmark, and Germany, began systematically preparing their citizens for combat—to become physically fit on behalf of their nations or, to put it another way, to weaponize the body in preparation for war. One of the fiercest proponents of this idea was Jahn, who founded the *Turnverein* (Turner) gymnastics club movement in the early nineteenth century. Jahn was a staunch military man who believed that physical education was the cornerstone not only of individual physical health but of national health, national identity—"somatic nationalism," as it's been called. This was not a new concept, of course—exercise had been incorporated into military training going back to Sparta in the eighth century B.C. and even longer before—but this was the immediate context in which Ling came of age.

LIKE JAHN IN Germany, Ling had always been "an intense patriot," according to the historian Fred E. Leonard, "eager to see his countrymen strong in body and soul and thus prepared to thwart the foe." Most of Sweden's southern and eastern Baltic provinces had been lost to Russia early in the eighteenth century, and now France, under Napoleon, threatened to take the entire country. Ling was driven to strengthen his country by helping strengthen and unify its citizens. Along with the work of Gutsmuths, Salzmann, and Jahn, he studied the latest in anatomy and physiology, a grounding in science that informed his philosophy on exercise, which, not unlike Mercuriale's, had a clear medical component at its core. Upon returning to Stockholm from Copenhagen in 1804, Ling, now twenty-eight, was determined to open an exercise training school inspired partly by Nachtegall's gym. This took several years, as he was developing his exercise techniques, but his proposal to the Swedish government was approved in 1813, and the following year the Royal Central Institute of Gymnastics—as it was named by the king—began operations.

Ling was given an annual salary plus funds to purchase some equipment and to rent space for the institute, which he led for the remaining twenty-five years of his life.

While Ling utilized some apparatuses in his classes—ropes, vaults, and so on—his primary innovation was in creating "free exercises" for both sexes that didn't require the use of equipment (partly for practical purposes, since equipment invariably had to be repaired or replaced). I found it difficult to imagine what Ling's idea of free exercise entailed, so I was particularly grateful that Lotta had arranged for me to view some rare, early film footage (preserved digitally) of students participating in Ling classes. Although the footage was taken nearly a century after the master's death, his regimens had been so precisely choreographed, notated, and described that they were apparently little changed from the time when Ling invented them. The best way I can think of to describe the "Ling Method," from what I have seen and read, is as a form of tightly choreographed calisthenics, incorporating body-weight exercises like push-ups and plank positions, synchronized dance steps, and vigorous, continuous movement—enough to accelerate the cardiovascular system—and performed in unison by large groups. Men and women attended classes separately, and all wore simple uniforms. Ling's calisthenics were, in a broad sense, a precursor to group fitness classes you'd find at just about any gym today, with at least one major exception: An insistence on *beauty* was a defining criterion of his work—the beauty to be seen, felt, and expressed when a mass of people move as one in precise, graceful, synchronized drills. This required a tremendous amount of practice and repetition—the same drills performed over and over again until each student performed so flawlessly that his or her individuality would be subsumed by the group and, figuratively, by the entire nation.

While understandable and even laudable on the face of it, a sinister side to this philosophy would later emerge. By infusing physical fitness with a spirit of extreme nationalism and demanding complete obedience to a single master directing training drills, Ling—together with his contemporary Jahn—inadvertently created a template for the gigantic group fitness programs that became emblematic of the Nazi Party, such as the League of German Girls and the Hitler Youth, antisemitic paramilitary organizations in the guise of wholesome exercise for identically uniformed boys and girls. Similar kinds of paramilitary exercise squads would also be found under totalitarian regimes in the Soviet Union, the People's Republic of China, and elsewhere.

On a far more positive note, Ling can be credited as among the first anywhere, at any time, actively encouraging exercise for women and children, and for helping bring PE classes to schoolrooms in both the United States and the U.K. From its inception, a primary mission of Ling's institute was to train instructors, male and female alike, who would go on to lead classes elsewhere, to spread the gospel of the Ling system, not only in Sweden but abroad, and indeed they did.

In 1877, a graduate of Ling's institute, Concordia Löfving, was appointed to the School Board of London as the city's first lady superintendent of schools, a groundbreaking position that allowed her to incorporate exercise classes into the curricula for schoolgirls. Löfving had been recruited from Stockholm for the simple reason that no English teachers were considered qualified for such a job. Five years later, Löfving was succeeded in the post by another Swedish graduate of Ling's institute, Martina Bergman-Österberg, a women's suffrage advocate who expanded physical education for girls to more than three hundred schools and made it part of her mission as lady superintendent to train other women to become PE instructors. Bergman-Österberg is also credited with introducing to the English school system "gymslips," sleeveless tunics designed to be loose, comfortable, and practical for girls to exercise in—an early example of athletic wear for women. As for Löfving, she went on to write *On Physical Education*, published in 1882, one of the first books by and for women on the subject of exercise.

Ling's influence extended to America as well. Just two years after his death in 1839, a gutsy-sounding entrepreneur who went by the name Madame Beaujeu (exact origin of the "madame" unknown) opened the first gym exclusively for women in Boston, and one in New York City four years later. Another notable American, Catharine Beecher, though defiantly not a suffragist—unlike her sister, *Uncle Tom's Cabin* novelist and women's rights advocate Harriet Beecher Stowe—nevertheless became a forceful advocate for women's exercise. As an educator and author, Catharine had studied Ling's approach to calisthenics, with its emphasis on gracefulness and continuous vigorous movement. Beecher wrote dozens of books for women, such as her *Treatise on Domestic Economy*, which was published in numerous editions across the 1840s and 1850s. Her book's title doesn't quite hint at its contents; it includes a chapter on "domestic exercises" designed specifically for women to do on their own at home (as opposed to having to attend classes or go to a gym), an antecedent to Jane Fonda's multiple innovations in the 1980s. Beecher even encouraged women to perform the exercises to music, "to serve as an amusement."

Certain men in America, influenced by both Ling and Jahn, became forceful advocates for exercise for women and children, too. One of the most well-known, Dioclesian (Dio) Lewis, taught, lectured, and wrote about the health benefits of exercise, with works such as the Ling-inspired *New Gymnastics for Men, Women, and Children* (various editions, 1862–68). Lewis also opened an influential school of physical education in Boston. It closed in 1868, but another school of Swedish gymnastics and physical education later opened in Boston with the support of two wealthy patrons, a Swedish-born aristocrat and Ling enthusiast, Baron Nils Posse, and a Boston philanthropist, Mary Hemenway. Ling's influence extended in the opposite direction globally as well—not via Sweden directly, but via the British Empire, and upon a distinctly Eastern discipline: yoga.

A FEW YEARS ago, much was made of the surprising rediscovery (by an intrepid grad student) of Walt Whitman's thirteen-part series, "Manly Health and Training," written under a pseudonym for the *New York Atlas* newspaper in 1858. Other than the fact of its existence—a long-lost, book-length series of opinion pieces on exercise, diet, health, and "manliness" by the famed American poet, which is indeed remarkable—I found the actual contents of Whitman's manifesto to be silly; certainly unscientific in parts (he still believed in the long-discredited theory of bodily humors); sexist in its focus on men and men alone; and, with its emphasis on eugenics, racist.

Far more important was a development that primarily took place across the Atlantic, also in the nineteenth century: the invention of the bicycle. Credit for this must go to a fairly long list of inventors who gradually improved its design and practicality, as historian David V. Herlihy has chronicled in his book *Bicycle*. The first verifiable claim for what is now called a "bicycle" (a term that was not introduced until the 1860s) belongs to a German baron, inventor, and civil servant, Karl von Drais, who invented his *Laufmaschine* (German for "running machine") in 1817. Drais conceived of his machine as an alternative to horses, which had become scarce at the time due to recent crop failures. His wood-framed machine—the first patented, two-wheeled, steerable, human-propelled vehicle—was intended not for exercise or recreation but for transportation—and emphatically meant for men alone. Its wheels were made of iron. The vehicle did not have pedals and a chain, like the bicycles of today; instead the rider propelled it forward by pushing off the ground with one foot, then the other, more like a scooter. Drais's mechanical horse soon became known by its inventor's name, a "draisine," or a "velocipede" (meaning "fast foot").

Variations of Drais's invention would follow over the next seventy-five years. Some were built with three wheels to make them more stable—tricycles—and some with four. Pedals were introduced—an advance over scooting along with your feet—but so too were extremely large, high front wheels paired with small back wheels, which meant your feet were far above the ground. Commonly known as "high wheels" or as "penny-farthings" (after two coins of different sizes, large and small), this model could be ridden at faster speeds than velocipedes—an obvious advantage—but was also less stable and more dangerous.

The real breakthrough didn't come until the 1880s, with the introduction of what became known as the "safety bicycle," so called for being safer to ride than the high wheelers they quickly replaced. Safety bicycles came with two spoked wheels of roughly equal size—short enough that a rider's feet could touch the ground—and closely resembled the bicycles we ride today. Along with the safer, faster, more streamlined design, the safety bicycle prompted a dramatic shift culturally in how bicycles were used and by whom. These were no longer considered dangerous toys just for men and boys—novelties, really—but increasingly as a legitimate form of transportation and recreation, and most radically, as suitable even for women to utilize. By the 1890s, a "ladies" version of the bicycle had been designed; it had a step-through frame, without the high horizontal bar linking back wheel to front, so that women could more easily mount and ride their bikes, and it could be purchased with a "skirt guard," which prevented long skirts and dresses from becoming entangled in the rear wheel and bike chain. The very parts such garments covered up in public (the glutes, quads, hamstrings, and calves) were those worked most strenuously in cycling—muscles most women had never had the opportunity to strengthen and develop as effectively before.

To my mind, it's not an exaggeration to say that this nineteenth-century machine, a bicycle designed specifically with ladies in mind, was one of the most significant advances to date in the history of exercise for women and girls worldwide. The link between these new female-friendly bikes and the burgeoning women's suffrage movement was undeniable, as the great American women's rights activist Susan B. Anthony so eloquently observed in 1896: "The bicycle has done more for the emancipation of women than anything else in the world. It gives women a feeling of freedom and self-reliance. I stand and rejoice every time I see a woman ride by on a wheel . . . the picture of free, untrammeled womanhood."

A Practice

Movement is the silent music of the body.

—WILLIAM HARVEY (1578–1657)

Just as class begins, a man rushes in and unrolls his yoga mat next to mine. It's the last spot left. His nervous energy, his anxiety, is immediately palpable. He struggles to catch up—pushing himself and getting frustrated. For a few minutes, I feel frustrated, too—I would move my mat if I could, but you can't do so easily, discreetly, in the yoga studio already crowded with seventy people. Instead, I make a conscious decision to change my mood. In his book *Problems*, Aristotle poses the question, "Why does the one associating with the person who is healthy not become healthier?" (whereas someone with an illness may make others sick). He has no answer. But I have come to believe that health in the broadest sense can be infectious. If I remain calm, for example, perhaps this will calm the nervous man next to me, too.

This Vinyasa class ("Power Yoga," it's called) at my gym in New York is challenging and fast. We first warm up with numerous repetitions of the basic flow—plank (inhale), chaturanga (exhale), upward dog (inhale), downward dog (exhale), repeat. The front of my mat is just inches from the front of the dimly lit studio. I can't see anyone behind me, including our instructor, Melinda, and before me there is only a neutral brown curtain to lose my gaze in. I might as well have my eyes closed as I am being led solely by Melinda's voice—her soft, melodic voice and her clear instructions, anatomically clear, every movement of every limb accounted for. I just listen, concentrate, and follow. I feel sort of like a character in a movie who has to disable a ticking time bomb while, over the phone, the chief of the bomb squad provides step-by-step instructions. But here, what we want, what we are trying to do with whatever tools we possess, is the opposite of disabling a tricky piece of machinery. Instead, yoga is about snipping the invisible wires within and making one *able*—able to do things with one's body that one might never have envisioned or thought possible.

Just last week, I did a Crow Pose for the first time. I had been practicing for about six months without much success. But on that evening, when I crouched, planted my hands on the floor, and positioned my knees atop my bent elbows, I found my balance immediately and, more important, felt no rush of fear. I found myself doing it. I held Crow pose for ten to twelve seconds, then got distracted by a thought, and fell back. I tried again. And again, I could do it.

With the class warmed up, Melinda begins leading us through increasingly complex positions. This is when we really start to sweat and the "power" in the class name becomes undeniable. I am amazed by her ability to lead such a large, diverse group (in age, gender, body types, experience, and ability) through sometimes highly challenging configurations of the body, step by step by step, without interruption, without hesitation—one position cascading seamlessly into another—and rarely if ever making a mistake, for instance, saying left hand when she means right.

At the same time that she is clearly directing us as a group, she is also paying attention to individuals. At one point well into the class, we are doing a bind while in a crouch, and she suggests that we might want to stand on one leg, while holding the bind, and move into a Tree Pose. I have done it before, though it's difficult—difficult to maintain one's balance, difficult to keep the bind, and difficult to have the strength to pull oneself up with the weight of one leg. I struggle, I fall, I struggle and keep trying. From across the room comes Melinda's voice: "Billy, not today—not today." And that is exactly the right thing to say. I'm not headed in the right direction, she can see, and the struggle is messing with my head. I look at Melinda and nod, then fold into child's pose, take a breath, move into plank, upward dog, and downward dog, and rejoin the flow.

I HAVE BEEN practicing yoga for a few years now, going to class once or twice a week and doing some at home. I had done yoga long ago—I remember taking a short course when I was in college in the early 1980s, and I took a class now and then during the time I lived in San Francisco—but I never pursued it seriously. Lifting weights was always my thing. What brought me back to yoga this time around was, to put it succinctly if crudely, a pain in the ass: I developed sciatica, inflammation of the sciatic nerve—a long, thick nerve that runs right under the pelvis bone and down each leg—from working at a desk, basically eight hours a day, for the past thirty years. Now, it hurts to sit. A match gets lit under my gluteus maximus. I have seen a neurologist. There is not a lot one can do about sciatica, except ease off one's seat and make changes to accommodate. Doing squats or leg workouts is out of the question for now, and I have had to create a makeshift standing desk—one small coffee table stacked atop another—for writing. But perhaps this is for the best. I am of an age when I should try to salvage whatever I can of my functioning body before everything goes south completely.

The yoga studio at my gym is on the fourth floor. It is noticeably warmer up here—the air ripe and humid both from the rising body heat of the floors beneath and from the collective breath emanating from the studio itself. It is also quieter—on this floor alone, no music is piped in over speakers. It draws the over-fifty crowd. Before yoga class started today, I nearly ran into a man my age pushing across the gym floor a tower he'd created from four step platforms (borrowed from the aerobics studio), topped by a forty-five-pound weight—the kind of back-to-basics exercise popularized by CrossFit, DIY-style. Back and forth, back and forth, he went—Sisyphean minus a mountain.

"That looks . . . really hard," I commented when the man came to a stop.

"Total body workout," he answered, between pants. "I do half an hour." He was red in the face and drenched in sweat, great drops of which marked his path, as if he'd been carrying a bottle of water with holes in it. I couldn't help but think of Friedrich Nietzsche: "One cannot just will; one must will *something*." He returned to his task with grim determination. I was happy to escape into the yoga studio.

What we practice here in New York—and, more generally, throughout much of the Western world—is different in innumerable ways from the various forms of yoga first practiced in India, where it originated. Which is not to suggest it is easy to trace the exact origins—and, as importantly, the originators, the inventors—of yoga. There seems to be a general consensus that yoga in its earliest form developed over five thousand years ago among the Indus-Sarasvati Civilization in northern India. It is first mentioned in print, albeit almost in passing, in the Rigveda, one of the four sacred texts of Hinduism, used by Vedic priests (Brahmans) and composed

between circa 1700 and 1100 B.C., confirming yoga's deep, historical roots within Indian spiritual practice and religion. Over time,
yoga—in both philosophy and practice—was refined by the
Brahmanas and the mystics of Hinduism who eventually documented their beliefs in the Upanishads, the sacred texts written in
Sanskrit, circa 800–200 B.C.

What is now known as the classical period of yoga bears the
influence of the mystic and yoga master Patañjali, who reputedly
wrote the *Yoga sūtras*, a foundational text on yoga theory and practice, at some point in the second century. I say "reputedly" because,
as with Aristotle and other ancient figures, there are unanswered
questions about whether Patañjali himself wrote the text or one or
more of his followers did. Regardless, the *Yoga sūtras* distilled the
practice of yoga into an "eight-limbed path" for reaching enlightenment, and Patañjali is often referred to as the father of yoga.

A few centuries after Patañjali, a significant shift took place as
yoga masters in India began to reject the more mystical teachings of
the ancient Vedas and instead place greater emphasis on the physical
body as a way to reach enlightenment. This form of yoga, called
Tantra, eventually evolved into Hatha yoga, the form most commonly
practiced in the West today.

In the late nineteenth century, yoga masters (yogis) from India
began to travel to the West to demonstrate and spread their teachings.
Among the most famous and successful was Swami Vivekananda,
who traveled and lectured widely in the United States, supposedly
wrote more than two hundred books, and established yoga centers
around the world. Interestingly, however, a migration from West to
East had an impact on yoga practice, too. This is where the Swede
Pehr Henrik Ling once again enters our story. Ling's mid-nineteenth-
century philosophy of exercise, which had been exported to Britain
via instructors trained at his Royal Central Institute of Gymnastics,
was also adopted by the British Army. British troops in turn inculcated

their Indian colonial subjects in Ling's system of mass group exercise. In part, this had to do with the fact that Ling's method required no apparatuses, no machinery, only the body, but other factors were also involved. The nationalistic spirit that had been central to Ling's and Jahn's conception of group exercise held appeal for the people of India as well and intersected with a burgeoning interest in their native form of exercise, yoga.

Yet another predominantly Western influence came into play in yoga's popularity: Near the end of the nineteenth century, regimens focused purely on physical fitness began to be swept up within a larger, global rise in what became known as "physical culture," a reaction to the advances of the Industrial Revolution. As labor became less physically demanding and people working in factories or similar settings became more sedentary, there was a surge of interest in exercise for men and women alike—voluntary physical exercise as a cure-all for the body, the mind, and even society itself. Health and fitness magazines for both sexes began to pop up at the turn of the century, such as the French photographer Edmond Desbonnet's *La Culture Physique*, Dr. Mortat's *La Culture Physique de la femme*, and American entrepreneur Bernarr Macfadden's *Physical Culture*. But the single most important figure in the worldwide physical culture phenomenon was a phenomenon unto himself, the Prussian-born bodybuilder, showman, and savvy businessman Eugen Sandow.

BORN IN 1867 as Friedrich Wilhelm Müller, a German Jewish name he later changed for the stage, Sandow left Prussia at age eighteen to avoid military service and traveled throughout Europe, often performing with circuses as a strongman. He was a natural: genetically gifted with a well-proportioned muscular build—comparable to the "Grecian ideal" captured in ancient sculpture, which he would later say had inspired him as a teenager—and driven and ambitious enough to perfect his body even more through weightlifting, with the hope of becoming a star. He eventually made his way to London, where he entered a British bodybuilding competition on a lark, easily beat the reigning champ, and in quick succession achieved national, and then international, fame.

Sandow capitalized on his popularity in novel ways over the course of his career. He wrote numerous books on exercise and body-building and published a magazine, *Sandow's Magazine of Physical Culture*. Performing as a strongman all over the world, he would pose and flex onstage, even traveling America at one point with the Ziegfeld Follies, billed as "The Perfect Man" and "The Unprecedented Sensation of the Century." But perhaps his most influential move was to open gyms and training schools under his name. Sandow was so well known a figure worldwide that his name would even appear several times in James Joyce's *Ulysses*, of all places. Leopold Bloom tells himself repeatedly that he "must" start doing "Sandow's exercises" again. Whether Bloom ever did resume them isn't entirely clear, but, regardless, Joyce provided a unique endorsement of Sandow's system in episode 17 of the novel:

> The indoor exercises, formerly intermittently practised, subsequently abandoned, prescribed in Eugen Sandow's "Physical Strength and How to Obtain It" which, designed particularly for commercial men engaged in sedentary occupations, were to be made with mental concentration in front of a mirror so as to bring into play the various families of muscles and produce successively a pleasant rigidity, a more pleasant relaxation and the most pleasant repristination of juvenile agility.

The term *bodybuilding* had been coined in 1881 by a young American physical culturalist, Robert J. Roberts, who worked for the Young Men's Christian Association (YMCA) in Massachusetts as an instructor in physical training. (Roberts may also be remembered as the inventor of the medicine ball.) But it was Sandow who made bodybuilding internationally recognized, popularized classic bodybuilding poses, and ignited interest in the pursuit—particularly by men, though not only by men—of a muscular body.

The relatively recent invention of photography played a major and often-overlooked role in Sandow's worldwide success. He was canny about using photography to show off his beautiful body—in his books, magazines, posters, signed photos, and so on. And he was utterly uninhibited about baring all. Simply seeing photographs of the handsome, mustachioed Sandow, posing naked in nothing more than a faux fig leaf to cover his genitals, makes it clear why he was such a sensation. Today, original Sandow photographs are highly sought after as collectibles.

In 1904 Sandow toured South Africa, India, and other parts of Asia. "As a businessman," Sandow's biographer, David Waller, observes, "Sandow was scoping out the enormous commercial opportunities of turning himself into a truly global brand. Like a colonial explorer, he sought to plant the flag of his exercise system in the virgin markets of Britain's imperial colonies . . . where he sought to replicate the success of his magazine and training schools." He was reportedly greatly irritated that Ling's system already had a foothold on the Indian continent. But Sandow held an enormous advantage, one he exploited brilliantly: Ling was long dead, whereas people could go see the sculpted and sexy Eugen Sandow in the flesh—even *feel* his naked flesh, his mountainous biceps, enormous thighs, and rippling abs. (He charged a fee for each feel, of course.)

Sandow's fame had evidently preceded him in India, where audiences in the thousands flocked to his shows. He was seen as a kind of fakir—almost a holy man—of the physical culture movement, who could "cure" the ill and disabled with his system of exercise. His muscular physique was unlike any commonly seen in India at the time, and yoga masters and followers—whose physical ideal until then had been, if not actual emaciation, something close—sought to emulate him and become "jacked," as we say today. "I was astounded at my reception," he later told the *Daily Mail*, "and the fact that I was so well known." The admiration went both ways; Sandow apparently fell in love with India, and he almost accepted an offer to stay there under the patronage of a Parsi businessman.

Now, what exactly is the connection between this entrepreneurial bodybuilder and yoga, other than mutual admiration between Sandow and yoga practitioners? Leading contemporary scholars, including the medical anthropologist Joseph Alter and the historian of yoga Mark Singleton, credit Sandow and the Indian "Sandow craze" with helping popularize yoga, which absorbed routines and poses associated with physical culture into traditional yoga practice. "Under the influence of Sandow," Singleton writes in his book *Yoga Body: The Origins of Modern Posture Practice*, "bodybuilding . . . enjoyed an unparalleled vogue in India from the turn of the century . . . [and] it was instrumental in shaping the 'indigenous' exercise revival from which modern postural yoga would issue." As Singleton puts it, "Yoga was conceived as a form of bodybuilding, and vice versa." I should add, however, that I have found no evidence that Sandow actually incorporated traditional yoga poses (say, *Vrksasana*, the standing "Tree Pose") into his strongman routines or, looking at it the other way, that yoga masters incorporated Sandow-style biceps flexing, for example, into yoga practice. Instead, it was the shared underlying philosophy—the focus on building a strong, fit, aesthetically pleasing, and healthy body—that linked the two, improbably, at a crucial moment in yoga's development.

MORE THAN A century after Sandow visited the country, I made a trip to India, my first: I spent six days in Mumbai, where I participated in a literary festival, and then a week on holiday in the far more rural Kerala region on the southwestern coast. On one of my first days in Kerala, I pushed myself out of bed just before seven A.M. and attended a yoga class near my hotel—the only time the class was offered. While I wouldn't for a moment try to generalize about yoga practice in India based on that single hour-long class, I can say that it was unlike any class I've ever taken anywhere before or since.

I was about five minutes late, both because I'd overslept and because I couldn't immediately find the entrance to the yoga center. I opened the screen door carefully so as not to make too much noise. The yoga master, a man of about seventy, registered my appearance with a disapproving glance. Then he brusquely grabbed a mat and tossed it in my direction. His disapproval was not unearned; I had shown disrespect by being late, I knew. Sitting beside the yoga master at the front of the studio was a very young girl.

I got myself settled quickly. There were only four other students there—that alone made it vastly different from the densely crowded yoga classes I've attended in the States. It was as warm inside the studio as it was outdoors—at least eighty-five degrees even at that early hour—"Hot Yoga," but without trendy branding or having to turn up a thermometer.

The yogi talked slowly, almost casually—and *talked* is the right word. It wasn't as if he were leading a class the way Melinda and many yoga teachers I've encountered in America do—insistent, rapid: *instructing*. This was not instructing—his tone was more one of informing. He just spoke, informing us of his knowledge, in a low-key voice. Early on, we sat with legs crossed and hands resting on our knees when he said, "Now, bring your thumb and middle finger to your nose . . . Close one nostril with your thumb . . . Breathe in slowly through the open nostril. Four seconds . . . Breathe out . . . Four seconds . . . Close the other nostril with your middle finger." And so on. That was it: a lesson in how to breathe with full concentration through one nostril at a time.

Nothing about the class felt remotely competitive, as yoga can seem at gyms and studios in New York. The pace was very slow, considered, as if there were no expectation that any one of us would get a pose or movement exactly right after he had explained and demonstrated it. Yoga is a lifelong pursuit, he implied; it takes time and devotion and—the key word—*practice* to master it.

However, there was at least one unexpected exception on that particular morning. The master's fourth or fifth instruction was to sit in the lotus position, inhale all your breath, suck your abdominal walls in as far as you can, and then roll your abdominal muscles from top to bottom as you exhale, sort of like a garage door going down, each section bulging as it rounds the corner, and then in reverse direction—the garage door going up. He pulled up his shirt to demonstrate; it was the kind of flashy move I could easily imagine Eugen Sandow doing.

I, along with the others, pulled my shirt up halfway to try. To my surprise, I did it on the first try, a consequence of having fairly developed abs, I suppose—or more likely, it was just beginner's luck—doing without thinking. I had no idea I had it in me. I looked up from looking up at my stomach, and the yoga master was smiling. "Look at that—you did it! It took me two weeks to learn how to do that." He chuckled lightly and smiled at me for the first time. "You are blessed."

The master led us through eight or ten more poses and breathing exercises. It was nothing I hadn't done before, but done here in a slower, simpler way. This wasn't meant to make you sweat. It was meant to stretch your limbs, focus and appreciate your breathing, understand your body's limits and potentials better, clear your mind.

As the class came to a close, the yoga master introduced the girl who had been sitting quietly beside him throughout: his nine-year-old granddaughter. With great pride, he explained that she, too, was a master—she had recently won a yoga competition at her school. She smiled shyly and bowed her head as her grandfather kept talking about her accomplishments. Someone in the class asked if she would show us. She demurred at first, and then, while her grandfather continued speaking, suddenly she popped into an amazing, acrobatic pose: balanced only on her forearms, her legs sprung up and over her head so that her feet hovered just in front of her upturned face. Someone gasped. Then she gracefully transitioned to a different pose: standing on one foot, she pulled her other leg all the way up behind her and over her head, so that it was as perfectly straight as her balancing leg. We applauded her, and she shyly resumed her seated position next to her fellow yoga master. "Namaste," her grandfather said quietly and bowed.

The Proof

What is Exercise? What does it do, and how does it do it?

—Archibald MacLaren,
A System of Physical Education, 1869

The very notion that exercise is *good* for you—for improving overall health and well-being—has been a presumption, even a truism, going back to ancient Greece and Rome, to the writings of Hippocrates, Plato, and Galen, as well as to ancient Egypt, China, and other cultures. The revered Indian physician known as Suśruta of India (ca. 800–600 B.C.) advocated exercise to maintain "equilibrium" in the body—and hence good health—and warned against excessive exercise. Not bad advice. And yet an ancient philosopher's or physician's thoughts on the topic, no matter how prescient, aren't really anything more than that: thoughts. Surprisingly enough, indisputable scientific evidence for the benefits of exercise was established only relatively recently. It was not until the early 1950s that a handful of scientists began investigating whether exercise actually contributes to lower morbidity and mortality rates in human beings.

One of the leading pioneers in this area was an unassuming British epidemiologist named Jeremy (or Jerry) Morris, a man who, after his death at age eighty in 2009, was called by some obituary writers "the man who invented exercise." That would be something of an exaggeration. A more accurate title for Dr. Morris might be "the man who invented the field of exercise science," although the truth is, he hadn't set out initially to study exercise at all.

Note Dr. Morris's profession: although trained as a medical doctor, he had become a clinical epidemiologist, one who had a particular interest in the social factors underlying public health issues. After World War II, one issue that emerged as an especially serious concern was a dramatic rise in coronary heart disease, which reached epidemic proportions in the U.K. As with lung cancer and peptic ulcer, the exact cause of coronary heart disease was unknown at the time. But Morris and his colleagues in the Social Medicine Research Unit—a British equivalent to a national public health agency—had a hunch that a person's *occupation* might somehow be a factor. Morris determined to study a cohort in a single field, one where different jobs were performed in distinctly different ways and, as importantly, where medical data on full-time employees would be readily available for study. In what now seems like an ingenious idea, Morris decided to focus on transportation workers—specifically, the drivers and the conductors of double-decker buses, trams, and trolleys. From 1949 through 1950, he studied about thirty-one thousand men (and as far as I can determine, it was exclusively men), ages thirty-five to sixty-four. Although the men worked in pairs in the same vehicle, their jobs were completely different: Drivers simply sat and drove all day, whereas conductors hopped off and back on the bus or trolley constantly and, in the case of double-decker buses, up and down the stairs countless times over their shifts. For these men, work itself was a workout.

Morris and his team scrutinized all available data: employees' absences of any duration due to illness; medical diagnoses obtained from general practitioners and hospital certificates; and details of all deaths, obtained via death certificates, and of retirements due to ill health. As for types of heart disease, the team looked specifically for cases of angina (severe pain in the chest, caused by inadequate blood supply to the heart and signaling further potential problems) and of coronary thrombosis (partial or total obstruction of an artery due to a blood clot), leading either to a nonfatal heart attack or to immediate death from a heart attack. The results were unambiguous. In Morris's paper on the study, first published in the *Lancet*, November 21, 1953, he concluded that the conductors—the men much more physically active on the job—had far less coronary heart disease than the sedentary drivers, and it appeared in them at a later age. Bus conductors did still have incidents of heart disease—however, primarily angina, a more benign symptom, and they had a far lower early mortality rate than the drivers they worked with. Among the thirty-one thousand transportation workers studied, immediate mortality from a heart attack was over twice as high in the drivers.

Morris's findings did not lead to an immediate link between exercise per se—voluntary exercise as we know it today—and better health and lower mortality rates. Confining his conclusions to the transportation study alone, Morris felt that it was "the greater *physical activity* of 'conducting'" that helped explain why these men remained healthier than their counterparts behind the wheel. Physical activity was the key determinant, and this helped establish a solid foundation for subsequent scientific research into exercise and heart disease and other ailments. However, Morris didn't stop there. His original findings prompted him to study the subject further. His next cohort: thousands of British postal workers and civil servants. As with the bus conductors and drivers, Morris found that postal workers who delivered mail by foot, walking miles a day and carrying loads of mail, had a far lower incidence of heart disease than their civil service counterparts, who worked in administrative roles, mostly sitting all day doing office work, paperwork, answering telephones, and so on.

Coincidentally, in 1953, the same year that Morris's initial report appeared in the *Lancet*, two New York–based experts in physical rehabilitation, Hans Kraus, MD, and Ruth P. Hirschland, published an academic paper on exercise that focused on an entirely different cohort: children, ages six to nineteen. About seven thousand children in the United States and abroad were studied, and Kraus and Hirschland found that American children fared less well—shockingly less well—than European children when given simple tests to measure their physical fitness, such as sit-ups, leg lifts, and toe touches. A more sedentary culture in America—dependent on cars and inclined toward sitting on the couch watching television—was blamed. The report didn't get much notice when it was first published. But when it reappeared the following year in the *New York State Journal of Medicine*, it came to the attention of John Kelly, a prominent Philadelphia financier and former national sculling champion (as well as the father of Grace Kelly). He was horrified by the findings that 56 percent of American children failed the simple fitness test, as compared with only 8 percent of the European children tested. He passed the report on to Pennsylvania senator James Duff, who convened a White House luncheon on the topic hosted by President Dwight D. Eisenhower.

Hirschland—by now divorced and going by Bonnie Prudden, an adopted nickname plus her maiden name—was invited to attend the luncheon along with a number of physical education experts and more than thirty leading professional athletes, such as Willie Mays and Bill Russell, thereby guaranteeing a significant amount of press coverage. Apparently, the vivacious and eloquent Prudden, in particular, made such a powerful impression on Eisenhower during the discussion that he directed Vice President Richard Nixon to convene a major conference and come up with a plan of action to improve the fitness of America's kids. This he did, and Nixon's conference led to the establishment in July 1956 of a new federal agency, the President's Council on Youth Fitness, which Eisenhower signed off on by Executive Order 10673.

Beyond the conferences held and high-profile influencers involved, there was one more factor—a highly personal one—that must have spurred President Eisenhower on to some extent: the year before, in 1955, he suffered a mild heart attack while in office. This came as something of a shock to the American public. Eisenhower, a fit-looking sixty-five and just two years into his eight-year term, was a five-star general and known to be a regular golfer. But he was also a smoker. And the cardiologist who oversaw his care, Dr. Paul Dudley White, warned the president to give up cigarettes and to exercise more regularly and vigorously. As Shelly McKenzie points out in her book on the rise of fitness culture in America, *Getting Physical*, "White's prescription for exercise flew in the face of traditional recovery plans [for a heart attack] that called for the patient's near immobilization for weeks after the incident and a long recovery at home." White's warning about cigarettes was ahead of its time, too. The first surgeon general's report on smoking and health, explicitly linking smoking to lung cancer and heart disease, did not appear until 1964.

While Eisenhower certainly deserves credit for establishing the Council on Youth Fitness, the truth is it failed to generate much publicity or interest during his administration. Eisenhower didn't go out of his way to promote it. That changed completely with the election of his much younger successor, forty-four-year-old John F. Kennedy, who expanded the council's aims to include adults as well as children and made promoting physical fitness a signature issue of his administration virtually from the start. Kennedy renamed it the

President's Council on Physical Fitness (PCPF) and spoke frequently on the topic, both to the media and in public. In a speech given in 1961, the year I was born, Kennedy cut right to the chase: "We are under-exercised as a nation; we look instead of play; we read instead of walk."

But it wasn't just talk. The new PCPF mounted a massive national advertising campaign to promote physical fitness and published a booklet, titled *Adult Physical Fitness*, with a series of simple routines for men and women—developed with input from dozens of experts—distributed free of charge to two hundred thousand households and sold for fifty cents or less to many thousands more. We had a copy in my house when I grew up; I remember it clearly, its patriotic red-white-and-blue coloring and the black-and-white photos of models demonstrating leg raises and step-ups. Looking through a copy now, I am amazed by how thorough and eminently sensible its prescribed exercise regimens for men and women are. The program begins with a warm-up; continues with "conditioning exercises," such as toe touches, push-ups, sit-ups, and leg raises; and concludes with a few minutes of "circulatory" activity, such as jogging, jumping rope, or running in place. With the exception of jogging, all exercises in the program can be performed at home without any equipment beyond a chair and your own body.

As laudable as the PCPF was (and still is—the council on fitness has evolved and expanded under succeeding presidential administrations), there is one thing glaringly missing from the promotional campaigns in its early years: people of color. The models in the PCPF booklet for adults are all white, as are nearly all models who appear in the PCPF posters and advertisements I've tracked down (occasionally a Black girl or boy is featured among groups of schoolchildren). Fortunately, there were African American–owned publishing companies, such as the groundbreaking Chicago-based Johnson Publishing, to help fill that gap. From the late 1950s and on through the 1970s and beyond, Johnson's popular magazines *Ebony* and *Jet* ran numerous articles on the importance of exercise for Black Americans, often featuring interviews with popular African American celebrities such as Dorothy Dandridge or Cab Calloway, who were pictured doing their own exercise regimes.

As for other communities of color in the United States—Latinos, Native Americans, Asian Americans—I've yet to find examples of comparable public health campaigns or major media coverage from that time period focused *specifically* on, and featuring images of, them. That would not begin to change until many years later. In fact, it was not until 1996 that the acting U.S. Surgeon General, Audrey F. Manley, MD (the second person of color, immediately following Joycelyn Elders, MD, to hold the position), issued a comprehensive "Report on Physical Activity and Health," backed up by years of scientific research into the topic. Addressing all Americans, Dr. Manley, a pediatrician particularly concerned by the rise in obesity, emphasized two simple points in her report: "First, demonstrated health benefits occur at a 'moderate' level of activity—a level sufficient to expend about 150 calories of energy per day, or 1,000 calories per week (e.g., walking briskly for thirty minutes each day). Second, although physical activity does not need to be vigorous to provide health benefits, the amount of health benefit is directly related to the amount of regular physical activity."

In retrospect, the ancients hadn't been too far off in their thoughts on exercise. As Plato put it more than two thousand years ago: "It is not the number of exercises but their moderate nature that brings about a good human constitution."

The Seventies

It is not necessary, as some may think, to be born strong in order to become strong. Unlike the poet who, we are told, has to be born a poet, the strong man can make himself.

—EUGEN SANDOW (1867–1925)

Virtually concurrent with the U.S. government's efforts to promote physical fitness back in the 1950s, another important influence was becoming deeply embedded in American culture: that would be television—the very medium blamed by some for turning Americans into underexercised couch potatoes. Enter Jack LaLanne, the trim, handsome, jumpsuit-wearing exercise evangelist, who began airing his groundbreaking exercise program, *The Jack LaLanne Show*, on a San Francisco TV station in 1951. Eventually picked up by ABC, it went nationwide as a daytime program in 1959 and ran until 1986, a few years after I had graduated college. His primary audience was women—often stay-at-home moms like my own, who would follow along from home as Jack did leg raises, jumping jacks, and sit-ups. Although there were other figures who either hosted local TV programs or appeared regularly on national talk shows to discuss and demonstrate exercises—Paige Palmer and Maggie Lettvin among them—Jack LaLanne was the true pioneer, in terms of using media to promote exercise, fitness, and weight loss. He was certainly part of my childhood, a man whose wholesome sexiness in that snug jumpsuit added to his telegenic appeal. Jack LaLanne was, for me, the 1960s version of Eugen Sandow. Ah, but then came the 1970s, my teenage years, and a whole new icon to replace him: Arnold Schwarzenegger, a figure who would also play a major role in changing the very reason for people to exercise.

It's hard for me now to dissociate the Schwarzenegger who became a conservative Republican and the governor of California from the Schwarzenegger who appeared seemingly out of nowhere in 1977. That's when the documentary *Pumping Iron*, on the subculture of male bodybuilding, was released and he began appearing in American magazines and on TV talk shows. It was like he'd come from another planet. (Actually, he'd come from Austria.) Arnold was sexy in an over-the-top, larger-than-life way, almost like an uber-masculine version of Marilyn Monroe. Over six feet tall, huge and handsome, "the Austrian Oak" had pecs bigger than any man's and a mischievous gap-toothed smile, suggesting he didn't take himself too seriously.

Arnold was so comfortable in his own skin—in his hypertrophied heterosexuality, as I would call it—that he didn't seem to mind at all being regarded as mere eye candy for men and women alike, straight and gay. Arnold did a nude centerfold for *Cosmopolitan*— granted, in a pose that tactfully hid his bits—but he also famously outdid Burt Reynolds by posing in an issue of *After Dark*, a mainstream performing arts magazine known to have a predominantly gay readership. Unquestionably meant to be homoerotic, these photos were pretty racy even by today's standards. Arnold, thirty years old and in his bodybuilding prime at the time, is shown naked in a locker room, as if he'd just stepped out of the shower, revealing his muscular bare buns in one photo and, in another, a clear glimpse of his penis.

The young Schwarzenegger was like Sandow—a shameless showman, exhibitionist, and entrepreneur—but Sandow on steroids. Like other bodybuilders of the period, and still today, his body was made hugely muscular and ripped, in part, by large doses of early forms of performance-enhancing drugs, such as Dianabol and Deca-Durabolin. It was an open secret, one that he admitted to publicly later in life. Whether male or female, you rarely get muscles like that without pharmaceutical help. In the 1970s, there were suddenly lots of big, handsome bodybuilders like Arnold out there—Franco Columbu, Lou Ferrigno, Serge Nubret, Frank Zane, to name a few— yet Schwarzenegger had something the others lacked and could not inject with a needle: movie-star charisma, as Hollywood would soon discover.

I saw *Pumping Iron* shortly after it first came out. I was sixteen years old, primed to be inspired by a bodybuilder with muscles as big as Schwarzenegger's. (My dad—though as athletic and into sports as ever—was never interested in lifting or spending time in his gym's weight room.) For my birthday, I asked my parents for a complete weight set, including a bench for presses, and began lifting daily in my bedroom, following regimens I found in my new favorite magazine, Joe Weider's *Muscle & Fitness* (which had been around, it turns out, since the physical culture era of the 1930s). Pretty quickly, I started to get more and more muscular. I tracked down Charles Gaines and George Butler's 1974 book *Pumping Iron: The Art and Sport of Bodybuilding*—a photo essay on Schwarzenegger and fellow competitors in a Mr. Olympia contest that had been the basis for the documentary—as well as a *Pumping Iron* calendar filled with beef-cake pinups. I imagine that, to my conservative Catholic parents, this new obsession with weightlifting served to confirm that their only son was 100 percent straight. Of course, it was the complete opposite. Let's just say that Arnold played a crucial role in my adolescent recognition that I was attracted to men.

At sixteen, I wasn't quite old enough (nor living in the right place) to really enjoy the seventies, that hedonistic yet somehow still innocent pre-AIDS period—"The 'Me' Decade," as Tom Wolfe famously named it in a 1976 essay—but I was certainly paying attention. There was a newfound sexual freedom in the air, thanks largely to the increasingly public rise of the women's liberation and gay liberation movements, with their emphasis on self-determination, liberty, and of course equality—under the law and in bed. Disparate cultural elements had also come into play in the loosening of sexual mores: the widespread availability of the birth control pill, for instance; the legalization of abortion in the United States; the mainstreaming of porn, as epitomized by the film *Deep Throat* (which came out in the same year—1972—as the more high-brow but still explicit *Last Tango in Paris*); and the success of slickly published, how-to erotica books, such as *The Joy of Sex* and *The Joy of Gay Sex*, which were unusually frank in explicating the pursuit of pleasure for its own sake, complete with elegant illustrations.

Exercise, bodybuilding, and health clubs, as some gyms began to market themselves, neatly fit into this "culture of narcissism," as the author Christopher Lasch called it in his 1979 book of the same name. As never before, being physically fit was unabashedly linked not just to healthfulness—which was almost a given by this point—but to sexiness: to be fit was to *be* sexy. How working out made you *look* was now as important, if not more important, than how it made you feel. As a personal fitness trainer once put it to me bluntly: "Let's face it: the main reason people exercise is to look good naked and get laid." For young men especially, Schwarzenegger, with his bronzed and oiled body like a gleaming trophy of sexual conquests, was a jacked-up embodiment of this idea. Getting pumped at the gym could even be as good as having sex: "It is the greatest feeling in the world," Schwarzenegger once said of the feeling he gets from working out. "A good pump is better than coming."

While Schwarzenegger had ignited my own interest in working out, there were a number of other tremendous athletes and exercise icons in the 1970s who emerged seemingly overnight during that pivotal decade—Bruce Lee, for example. He did for martial arts what Schwarzenegger had done for bodybuilding. Lee's incredible athleticism; lean, rock-hard physique; and unprecedented martial arts skills—captured in hugely successful films such as *Fist of Fury* (1972) and *Enter the Dragon* (1973)—started a craze for the various East Asian martial arts that had till then hardly existed in the West, a craze that continues to this day in the popularity of mixed martial arts and the UFC league. Just as significantly, the Chinese American Lee, who died at the terribly young age of thirty-two, helped change the way Asian men in general were seen, defying retrograde stereotypes of submissiveness or weakness. To the contrary, he was a peerless fighter, as supreme an athlete and just as tough as his contemporary, the boxer Muhammad Ali.

In other sports, mustachioed Mark Spitz literally and figuratively became the poster boy for swimming after winning seven gold medals at the 1972 Olympics. In his red-white-and-blue Speedo—an image as ubiquitous as the poster of Farrah Fawcett in a red swimsuit would be a few years later—he made swimming seem sexy and cool. The affable Frank Shorter, a surprise Olympic gold medalist in the marathon that same year (and a silver medalist in 1976), is credited with popularizing jogging and long-distance running as never before; somehow, he made running twenty-six miles look easy. From there, the running and jogging phenomenon quickly became a whole new industry—running shoes, shorts, and other gear, magazines, and even books, as exemplified by the success of Jim Fixx's 1977 bestseller *The Complete Book of Running* with its striking cover image of the author's muscular legs, caught midstride, against a bright red background.

WITHOUT QUESTION, THERE were a number of celebrated, highly gifted female athletes at the time who inspired women and men alike, too—the American runner Mary Decker, the gymnasts Olga Korbut of the Soviet Union and Nadia Comăneci of Romania, and tennis greats such as Billie Jean King and Martina Navratilova, to name a few—but I would propose that it was neither a man nor a woman who made the most substantive, long-lasting impact on women and girls' lives when it came to exercise and athletics in the late twentieth century. Instead, it was a piece of legislation, signed into law in the United States on June 23, 1972, called simply Title IX.

It is crucial to understand, and to remember, that Title IX was enacted as an addition to the Civil Rights Act of 1964, which was intended to end discrimination in employment and "public accommodation" based on race, color, religion, or national origin. A parallel law, Title VI, signed into law by President Lyndon Johnson in 1964, prohibited discrimination in federally funded private and public entities based on race, color, and national origin. But Title VI did not include discrimination based on sex, and activists involved in the women's liberation movement of the early seventies, in particular, began to lobby Congress to add sex as a protected class category.

In legislation coauthored jointly by Congresswoman Patsy Mink of Hawai'i (the first woman of color and first Asian American woman elected to Congress) and Senator Birch Bayh of Indiana, Title IX, signed into law by President Richard Nixon, was designed to fill this gap. The heart of the law—a single sentence—reads like simplicity itself: "No person in the United States shall, on the basis of sex, be excluded from participation in, be denied the benefits of, or be subjected to discrimination under any education program or activity receiving Federal financial assistance."

Note that it doesn't single out women; the law applied to women and men alike. (Under the Obama administration, the statute was interpreted to safeguard against discrimination on the basis of gender identity and transgender status as well. In early 2017, the Trump administration dismantled key protections for transgender people, but thankfully this was reversed by Executive Order under President Biden.) Nor was Title IX solely a so-called sports-equity law, as some have understandably misperceived it. The bottom line is, Title IX was applicable to *any* federally funded public educational program, including science, technology, and mathematics programs. Even so, it is chiefly known today for changing how women and girls could participate in sports and athletic programs in American high schools and colleges, if only by providing equitable funding and equal opportunities for them. It also marked a sea change in long-held stereotypical views of what had once been called "the weaker sex." Now girls could aspire to be not only gymnasts, figure skaters, and tennis players but also basketball, baseball, soccer, volleyball, martial arts, boxing, and hockey stars.

But of course, it didn't happen overnight, and Title IX wasn't passed without controversy. Some claimed—and continue to claim— that the added protection for girls came at the expense of athletic programs for boys at both the high school and collegiate levels. (Wrestling, a prototypically male sport, is often mentioned as having been a victim of lost funding and stature as a result of the new law.) While it is true that some programs for young men were cut or cut back in some areas in order to address the inequitable opportunities for girls, I see this as a necessary and long overdue balancing of the scales. And research shows that there *has* been a substantial increase in female athletic participation over the past fifty years. One study published in 2006 showed that the number of women in high school sports was nine times larger than it had been in 1972, while the number of women in college sports had increased by almost 500 percent over that time.

Now, one may logically ask, what is the actual, historical link between the advances wrought by Title IX and participation by women and girls in various forms of exercise? After all, I've never maintained that organized sports or athletic competition and exercise are the same thing. But I would argue that Title IX effectively hit the reset button culturally, politically, legally, and even financially in the United States, opening up opportunities for women to sweat—really sweat—as much as the other sex. What better example is there than Jane Fonda?

FONDA, WHO WAS born in 1937, points out in her autobiography, *My Life So Far*, that she had "entered so-called adult life at a time when challenging physical exercise was not offered to women." In the 1950s and 1960s, "We weren't supposed to sweat or have muscles." She had studied ballet for twenty years; that was her way of staying in shape. But that changed when she fractured her foot while filming *The China Syndrome* in 1978. She could no longer don toe slippers and take ballet classes, yet, at age forty-one, she was determined to get really toned and lean for a role in her next film, *California Suite*, in which she would have to appear in a bikini in one scene. Fonda's stepmother suggested that she try a class at the Gilda Marx studio in Century City once her foot had healed. Apparently, there was a "marvelous" teacher there named Leni Cazden.

As Fonda describes it, Cazden's class was not as physically vigorous as the aerobics classes that would become the rage in the 1980s, thanks largely to Fonda herself; it was more of a low-impact conditioning class, similar to what you'd see demonstrated on Jack LaLanne's TV show or what was prescribed by the President's

Council on Physical Fitness. But there was at least one distinct difference: the music. Cazden played a mix of pop and R&B songs throughout her classes: Fleetwood Mac, Teddy Pendergrass, Stevie Wonder, Marvin Gaye. Fonda loved it. "I began to move to a different rhythm, becoming one of those people you see through their car windows singing and grooving to music only they can hear," she writes. "I never did go back to ballet." Fonda, who considered herself a "recovering food addict," and who also suffered from bulimia for many years, now became "addicted" to Cazden's exercise classes: "I hated to miss even a day." When there were no scheduled classes, Fonda would hire Cazden to teach her privately.

Going into the exercise business was not an idea born purely out of Fonda's newfound love for exercise. Her husband, the political activist and future California state congressman Tom Hayden, had recently created a grassroots organization called the Campaign for Economic Diversity (CED), a statewide nonprofit focused on economic equality, renters' rights, environmental protection, and related issues. As with many nascent nonprofits, funding the CED was a serious challenge from the start, and Hayden and Fonda had been brainstorming for months about different ways to raise money. They had considered opening a restaurant or an auto repair shop— businesses they knew nothing about, Fonda notes—and then one day it hit her: Exercise was something she had become passionate about. She'd partner with Leni and open a workout studio. Leni liked the idea, they came to an agreement and found a small studio space in Beverly Hills, and the two women opened the doors to Jane and Leni's Workout in 1979. Under the terms of the agreement, the business would be owned by the CED, with profits going directly toward supporting the organization. This meant that Fonda herself wasn't going to make a dime (at least in the beginning). Cadenza, like other employees—teachers, a managing director—would be paid a salary.

"We weren't at all prepared for the huge success," Fonda recalls in her book. From day one, "it was like an avalanche, without our once having to pay for advertising." Due to the Oscar winner's celebrity, "Talk show hosts Merv Griffin and Barbara Walters *asked* to come and film classes. People flocked from all over the country." It became, in her words, "a worldwide phenomenon, beyond anything any of us had ever imagined." And this was while they still ran just one studio.

They began developing a host of new workouts to keep their clients, mostly women, coming back to try different classes, many of which Fonda herself led: Beginning, Middle, and Advanced workout classes; Pregnancy, Birth, and Recovery workout classes; stretching classes; classes for menopausal women; and classes with different types of music—pop, disco, country, and so on. Fonda, together with Cazden and their instructors, was developing a whole new vocabulary for exercise—and, whether she realized it or not, *material* for a range of books and videos. She studied anatomy and physiology, she has said, and became conversant in the basics of exercise science, including aerobic exercise.

Just over ten years earlier, in 1968, the American physician Kenneth Cooper had published his pioneering book, *Aerobics* (a term that was virtually unknown to the public at the time), which explained the benefits of aerobic exercise—continuous, low- to high-intensity exercise that raises the heart rate and increases oxygenation to the body's largest muscles, generally requiring fifteen to twenty minutes of strenuous activity. Cooper's original book resembled a fairly dry scientific text. But in 1979, the same year Fonda was opening her studio, he published a revised version geared to a mass market, *The New Aerobics*, which provided a simple point-system for tracking your aerobic activity through walking, running, and other simple cardio activities. The stars had aligned: The worldwide craze for aerobics had begun.

Two years later, in 1981, Fonda wrote *Jane Fonda's Workout Book*, which remained on the *New York Times* bestseller list for two years. A series of other best-selling exercise books followed. But it was her risk-taking foray into videotapes that made working out for women, in particular, revolutionary—and made millions of dollars.

Fonda says that she had to be convinced to make her first video in 1982. At the time, virtually no one owned a VCR; they were expensive, and there wasn't a market for commercial videotapes. Fonda herself didn't have a VCR, and as an actor, she wondered if a cheaply produced video would damage her film career, make her look "foolish." A businessman named Stuart Karl had proposed the idea to her, having been persuaded by his wife, who had read Fonda's *Workout* book. It took Karl several tries before Fonda said yes; she only hoped it might make a little more money for the CED.

The first video, *Jane Fonda's Workout*, went on to become one of the most successful home videos of all time (reportedly, more than seventeen million copies have been sold, raising so much money for the CED that Fonda eventually changed the original business arrangement, so she became sole proprietor of the multimedia workout business). The "home" in that phrase *home videos* was key: Women didn't have to join a gym or hire a babysitter to watch the kids when they wanted to work out; didn't have to travel to Fonda's studio in Beverly Hills; didn't have to go outside for a walk or run. They could "do Jane," as it became known, in the privacy of their homes, whether in Ohio, South Africa, or Guatemala, and wearing whatever they wanted. Fonda, an exceptionally effective teacher, led you through numerous stretching exercises to warm up, then moved into what I would call a medium-intensity cardio workout, performing simple exercises for every part of the anatomy—arms, shoulders, abs, and so on—all the while cheering you on with genuine enthusiasm. "Lift, release, squeeze it tight!" she called out while demonstrating an exercise for the buttocks. "Work *deep*! Five, six, seven, eight—*go* for the burn!" The main workout was followed by a cooldown that incorporated gentle yoga poses.

All these years later, Fonda's original workout, now available online, holds up remarkably well. Of course, back when the video came out, the only way to view it was on a VCR, but partly driven by the success of Fonda's *Workout*, that market exploded, and the machines became more affordable. The video itself was relatively inexpensive—far cheaper than a gym membership—and new versions came out regularly. At last count, Jane Fonda had made twenty-three exercise videotapes and twelve audio programs, in addition to her many workout books.

With the multiple advances in the seventies and early eighties, the foundation was now firmly in place: Fitness was poised to become the diverse, multibillion-dollar global industry it is today. And yet, right at this very moment, this turning point in the history of exercise, a world-changing, life-killing agent began to surface—a virus that has taken more than thirty-two million lives to date.

The Men in the Mirrors

Life is but a motion of Limbs . . .

—THOMAS HOBBES, *LEVIATHAN,* 1651

I
t is difficult now to call up the particular mood that prevailed in the AIDS pandemic's early years. I am not talking about the first rumblings, in the early 1980s, when no one knew enough to be afraid, but further in. In those post-AZT drug days before protease inhibitors, there was very little one could do if infected. Primitive prophylaxes against certain opportunistic infections offered one's best bet, but certainly no guarantee that one wouldn't die of Kaposi's sarcoma or cytomegalovirus or Pneumocystis carinii pneumonia. The idea of people with AIDS still being alive in thirty or forty years was almost unimaginable.

I had moved from Seattle to the Castro, as if to another country, in July 1985, right at the time when Rock Hudson died and every newspaper was filled with stories about the deadly virus. I was twenty-four. I had come out to my family after graduating college a year before, though I'd been sexually active since I was a teenager.

When I told my father I was moving to San Francisco, ground zero in the pandemic, he said he thought I might as well commit suicide. But I was ecstatic to be at the center of it all, living in a ratty flat off Diamond Street with four roommates, three cats, and a spectacular view of the city.

It was not illness or exposure to HIV I feared most at the time, but the disappearance of men I did not know. Someone I would see often at the gym or on the bus, or a man I would purposefully look for at the Stud, returning week after week and hoping to meet him, was suddenly missing. Of course, he could have moved, received a job transfer, or joined a new gym. He could have been hit by a bus, I would remind myself. But I learned quickly that the lottery-logic of most people's lives did not apply there. It was as if Oscar Wilde's aphorism—"It's an odd thing, but anyone who disappears is said to be in San Francisco"—had been updated and darkly inverted.

Terribly familiar with the strange new illness, some men I knew seemed able to sense it from blocks away, like the city's changeable weather—even in the earliest stages, when only the new HIV antibody test provided proof. It was "that look," they called it, nothing more. Their intuition fascinated me, until I shared it. After a couple of years and a couple of friends' deaths, I acquired this skill, too.

It was the predictability of the plotline, not the disappearing characters, that gradually became most frightening. Every time one story abruptly ended, another instantly started—on a loop. I remember that my friend Peter had just died when I visited another friend, Jeff, to bring him some food. Jeff was twenty-four years old. He had just been released from the hospital. In pain from persistent headaches and weakened by diarrhea, Jeff had staged a suicide attempt in his doctor's waiting room so that he would be admitted to the hospital on the spot, without several hours' delay. "I took just enough to faint— only pills," Jeff had explained to me. "You have to take more—and alcohol—to do it all the way." He knew what he was talking about:

Like many gay men at the time, he was a member of the Hemlock Society, which advised people about methods of suicide.

Now he was staying with Stuart, who had what was then called ARC (AIDS-related complex) and was in the midst of a widely publicized hunger strike to protest the meager federal AIDS funding under President Ronald Reagan. This was the winter of 1986. Opening the front door to their apartment was like cracking open an oven turned to 450 degrees. I immediately began unpeeling layers of clothing. Stuart was propped on the couch between two plump older men, wrapped in a sleeping bag, shivering, only his blond hair, emaciated face, and wire-rim glasses visible. The room was lit by a collection of seven or eight electric space heaters that crackled, hissed, and wheezed, bursting on and off, and cast a warm orange glow on the floor. No one spoke a word. The only thing on the wall was a giant calendar, marking Stuart's hunger strike countdown, covered with Xs. The door had disappeared behind me in the darkness.

Standing there, I felt for one delirious moment the final terror of illness: horribly, inescapably trapped, just like Jeff and Stuart— trapped in life, in a body unready to die, and desperate to jump out of it. I thought, if I join the other two men quietly waiting their turn on the couch, if I make myself at home here, I will never leave this apartment. I found my way to the kitchen, placed the food in the empty refrigerator, and then looked in on Jeff, who was sleeping. The last image I have of him alive is in that dim, hothouse bedroom. In spite of the heat, he was sprawled diagonally atop the bed, face down, wearing a hat, gloves, and a winter coat, as if he had fallen in knee-high snow and couldn't get himself up again.

A couple of days later someone found him dragging a bucket of water and a space heater around the apartment, searching for an electric socket. Jeff had to go back into the hospital, where he was forced to participate in group therapy and, thought to be suicidal, undergo a battery of psychiatric tests. The doctors could not find anything wrong with him. He stopped talking after several days in the ward, I was told. I remember thinking, I'm not surprised: He is ready to die, and he doesn't want to talk about it to anyone—whether doctor, social worker, or friend—anymore. I interpreted his silence as a noble surrender. It wasn't until an autopsy was performed that doctors discovered lesions on Jeff's brain, due to AIDS, which caused his loss of speech and dementia.

FACES OF THE dead surfaced weekly in the *Bay Area Reporter*, a local gay newspaper that published obituaries with photos of men who had recently died of AIDS. Picking up a copy, I would instinctively open first to this section; it filled two pages or more. I always recognized someone I had known, someone I had danced, slept, or worked out with, aware that, in a barely different narrative, one of the pictures could have been my own.

For a while, I saved the obituaries and other ephemera from—that is, evidence of—the pandemic: ACT UP meeting agendas; a Polaroid photo, passed among friends, of KS symptoms; a flyer that simply said, "Imagine a Cure"; a gay-paper personals ad that proposed, "Will Trade AZT for Seconal." As an HIV-negative gay man, I suppose that I felt a sense of duty to be an archivist of sorts for my community. Yet when I fell in love with Steve, I threw the yellowing papers away. Keeping up with every treatment-of-the-month seemed a daunting task, and the fattening files in our bedroom only served to remind me of the burgeoning death tolls, upon which I was determined not to dwell. This was in 1989. The worldwide pandemic was more than a news story now. It was in my house, in Steve's body, in our life.

One night I dreamed that Steve and I were knocking at a friend's door. He answered.

"Hello," I said tentatively, unsure what tone to strike. "So, we heard that you are well. That you don't have it anymore."

"Yeah," he replied calmly. "Now I'm just trying to live without it."

We all laughed nervously.

"Well, what did you do?" Steve asked. "What did you take? Who's your doctor?"

He started to answer, but someone called to him from within the house. "Sorry, I'll be back in a minute," he promised. "Wait here."

Steve and I waited and waited. The friend never returned.

Our waking life often had the quality of that dream: We stood together, supported each other, sure that the answer would come, but skeptical, too, tired of waiting.

That it *did* actually come one day—in the form of protease inhibitors, around 1996 or so, and for Steve, in the nick of time—never failed to seem miraculous. After four or five years, Steve had regained his lost health—his T cells steady and "viral load" now undetectable—and we, like so many with access to these drugs, breathed more easily. But there was never a sense of complacency, of forgetting. How could there be? For his part, Steve had to take the pills on a strict schedule every day, had to switch medications from time to time, cope with side effects, get blood work regularly, and so on. For mine, I was always acutely aware that, with one unsafe slip or accident, I could find myself on a drug cocktail, too.

Before Steve, I had never pictured myself in a long-term relationship. Lovers, sex, romance—yes—but to pair off with one person and make a life together? No. And then, because of AIDS, I never presumed that our relationship would last long enough to be truly long-term. What I got so unexpectedly, however, I also unexpectedly lost.

THE EVENING BEFORE Steve died, we had gone to the gym together. To this day, I can still picture him doing sit-ups and other ab exercises in the stretching area while I moved on to lift weights. I don't know why that image, that scene, still plays on a loop in my head three decades later—but it does. Maybe it's because he looked so healthy, so fit—only to be gone the next day. Maybe it's because Steve and I had first met at a gym more than sixteen years before: the ending and the beginning of our relationship fusing in one moment—on a gym floor.

That gym, now long gone, too, was called Muscle System. It was not "a gym" but *the* gym for gay men in San Francisco at the time. Muscle System was a "men only" gym—and by *men*, I mean, in this instance, gay men, with just a few straight exceptions. It was known as a gay gym, pure and simple, an institution that went extinct at some point in the last two decades. (Back then, some referred to Muscle System, whether homophobically or affectionately, as "Muscle Sissies.") I don't know if the gym actually enforced it—prohibited or prevented or intimidated women from joining—but I am quite sure I never saw a woman working out there in my fifteen years as a member.

Every wall of Muscle System—a skylighted, two-level space—was lined with floor-to-ceiling mirrors, providing a perfect stage for studying yourself from a variety of perspectives. Sure, there were always die-hards who worked out intensely, but Muscle System was never really a hardcore bodybuilding gym, like Gold's. Anyway, for most gay men at the time, whether or not we were HIV-positive (and more than half of us in San Francisco were in those days), "body-building" during the AIDS era went beyond athletics or simple narcissism. It was no longer just about looking good and getting laid. Working out pitted us in direct competition not only with age but with AIDS. When a guy said he "should get in shape," it may have been to fight the virus or to stave off wasting syndrome (a common side effect of AIDS), not simply to get a boyfriend or to lose some weight. For someone else, gaining mass, losing fat, and strengthening muscles demonstrated measurable control over his body at a time when he might otherwise feel helpless about the virus slowly damaging it, or about the toxic drugs ingested to fight such a deadly disease.

If nothing else, muscles could make a man *look* strong, healthy, and attractive, even if he didn't feel that way inside. At Muscle System—where some men actually pumped up at home first, just to look good from the moment they walked in the door—a great body could be the best defense against sexual rejection and the secret of having HIV.

There was often more talking than weightlifting going on when the gym was full. It was not at all uncommon for locker-room gossip to mix seamlessly with the latest on HIV. Between sets, one might hear a group of lean young men discussing last night's AIDS benefit before turning to the finer points of the Mr. Leather contest and nipple piercing. Near the water fountain, two friends might be heard making plans to bring food to another gym member, at home with an oxygen tank and a prescription for morphine. The gym rarely provided a complete respite from AIDS, a chance to forget entirely; there simply was no spot in the city that did. Even the ubiquitous ACT UP T-shirts and music blaring throughout—like Neneh Cherry's AIDS-inspired reconstruction of "I've Got You Under My Skin"—occasionally served as grim reminders of the mess we were in.

As if we needed it. Directly or indirectly, every gay man was in some stage of the disease—infection, illness, survival, caregiving, denial, or mourning. Indeed, the degree to which AIDS was central to our lives may have been best expressed *at* the gym, where night after night the rotating members of the club came together: healthy, fresh-faced arrivals to the city constantly replacing those who'd left it. At Muscle System's front desk, notes taped to the counter occasionally announced memorial services for fellow gym members and employees who had died. The notes often showed up before the obituaries appeared in that week's *Bay Area Reporter*.

I remember seeing one about a memorial for Mark, a congenial thirty-two-year-old southerner who had made his entrance after work nearly every night for years. Although I never really knew him, I noticed when Mark was there, and his absence if he wasn't. Always impeccably dressed in a suit, tie, and full-length camel-hair or trench coat, with briefcase and gym bag in hand, he would throw a towel around his neck and sail to the locker room, waving "Hallo, halloo" to everyone in his path, adding each man's name if he remembered it.

When I'd last seen him at Muscle System about six weeks before, he appeared to have lost fifteen or twenty pounds—not an unusual sight in San Francisco at the time, although more likely due to AIDS than to exercise and dieting. I never saw him again. How could someone so young and energetic have gone so quickly? How could he, too, be lost? It was as if one day at the gym—working out, as always, in fluorescent bike shorts and a tank top—he simply walked right through the mirrors and disappeared.

A Break

Exercise should cease as soon as the body begins to suffer.

—Galen, *The Art of Medicine*, ca. a.d. 180

S ometimes it's good to take a break from exercise, as I'd learned in my fitness training course—give your joints, tendons, and ligaments a rest, and your mind as well. But sometimes a break lasts far longer than you had planned or ever imagined. This was my story for a while. I took a break both from exercising so much and from working on this book. And when I say I took a break, I'm not talking about weeks. I'm talking about years.

This whole phase, this breakup that exercise and I had, started not long after I lost Oliver, who died at eighty-two in August 2015. We used to swim together two or three times a week—usually a mile-long swim at a nearby pool—sharing a lane and often splitting a weekly session with a swim coach. We swam wherever we could—in cold mountain lakes, in salty seas, and in New York's overchlorinated public pools. We swam at elegant hotels in London and Iceland, Jerusalem and San Francisco. We went scuba diving in

Curaçao and St. Croix. One of the funniest memories I have is of swimming with Oliver in the huge public pool in Central Park on a steamy hot summer night—so hot that the pool was jammed with swimmers, kids, families, New Yorkers. The few lifeguards on deck were frantically trying to impose some order, keeping boys from cannonballing or dive-bombing, their whistles blaring above the din. But it was a lost cause, more like swimming in Times Square. And there in the middle of it all was Oliver, half-blind but indomitable, trying to do laps as I swam right beside him, his stressed-out bodyguard.

Oliver continued to exercise up until nearly the very end of his life—still swimming, albeit more slowly and at shorter distances. When he could no longer safely walk to the gym to work out, his trainer, a lovely guy named Ian, came to the apartment and took him through a cycle of simple exercises using light dumbbells, stretch cords, and a Bosu ball. For some cardio, he'd stride up and down the corridor. Even when confined to bed, he made a point of moving his limbs this way and that as vigorously as he could. "Exercise for the dying," Oliver sardonically called it. But he did it because exercise made him feel good, made him feel alive.

We held Oliver's memorial at the New York Academy of Medicine's auditorium, where the stage was filled with hundreds of fresh ferns—his favorite species of plant. Afterward, we had a reception in the gallery space just down the hall from the Rare Books room, the very place where I had first encountered Girolamo Mercuriale and *De arte gymnastica*. It felt comforting somehow.

Once Oliver was gone, though, all went silent, life became very quiet, and my interest in exercise went silent, too. None of it mattered much to me, suddenly, including exercise's history. It all seemed quite trivial, quite unimportant. I put this book aside and did not even open up the file on my computer for almost four years. In the interim, I wrote a different book, a memoir about my life in

New York and with Oliver, and published a volume of my street photography.

Single, alone, bored, depressed, I also began hanging out at a neighborhood pub on many nights, drinking more than I should, and on weekends, smoking more weed than I could justify. I still got some exercise, in a desultory way, now and then—but I'd lost my passion for it. As extra pounds accumulated where a six-pack had once been, my will weakened tenfold. The gym or the pool or a yoga class seemed like increasingly far-off destinations. Then, early in 2018, I was diagnosed with high blood pressure. This wasn't unexpected—three of my five sisters also had it, as did my late mother—and my blood pressure had always run a bit high. My doctor prescribed medication, but also this: "You need to step up your cardio."

"Right. I thought you'd say that."

At age fifty-seven, I faced a new reality: What had once been a choice no longer was, in that exercise changed from something I freely wanted to do—to look good, to feel good—to something I really should do to stay healthy. No excuses.

It took time, but exercise and I reunited, one might say, albeit in a different way. Since Oliver's death, coming just nine years after Steve's, I had changed. I felt like a different person, and hence exercise had changed for me, too. My feelings were not those of the obsessiveness of youth, but more like a civilized arrangement between former lovers, now well into middle age. I resumed working out and swimming regularly, and as a result my blood pressure returned to normal, my weight dropped, and, by my fifty-ninth birthday in January 2020, I felt better than I had, physically and mentally, in a long time.

And then the pandemic hit.

In mid-March, the governor shut down all gyms in the state (along with many other measures) to prevent the spread of the coronavirus. The same was true in cities all around the world—gyms closing virtually overnight, a whole industry, not to mention a way of life for millions, suddenly ending. This was not the first time that gyms had been forced to close in response to a public health crisis. During the flu pandemic of 1918, which ultimately claimed at least half a million lives in the United States alone, chapters of the YMCA were closed for months at a time to prevent the spread of that deadly virus; indoor sporting events were banned; and people were encouraged to get exercise (and children to play games, nicknamed "flu games") outdoors. Similarly, at the height of the polio epidemic of the early 1950s (far smaller by comparison to the 1918 flu and Covid-19 pandemics), swimming pools were closed because the poliovirus—an enterovirus that enters the body through the intestinal rather than the respiratory system—can be transmissible through water contaminated with traces of fecal matter. (In retrospect, the polio pool closures were something of an overreaction, as few cases were actually traced to swimming pools.) Yet these precedents paled by comparison to the fallout from Covid-19. By the end of 2020, as the country approached the grim milestone of five hundred thousand deaths in less than a year, at least 15 percent of gyms in the United States had closed permanently, according to the International Health, Racquet and Sportsclub Association, with the full scope of gym closures and related bankruptcies still unknown.

Like everyone else during the pandemic, I had no choice but to adapt when my gym closed. I developed a twenty-minute home exercise routine: push-ups, chin-ups, standing squats, sit-ups, some yoga, and I made a point of going for a walk almost every day. I never did go the virtual route—following trainers' workouts on Instagram Live or Zoom, or doing yoga classes via YouTube—nor was I interested in high-tech fitness machinery like Peloton or the Mirror (not that I could have afforded them anyhow). I remember seeing a TV ad for the Mirror and finding it very strange—futuristic, but not in a good way: people energetically working out by themselves while watching themselves in front of a personal trainer visible virtually in a full-length mirror. A high-tech version of Narcissus for the rich. It seemed to me to epitomize how disconnected people had become and may want to remain from now on—so different from the AIDS era: everyone at home alone, isolated, safe in their sanitary mirrored pods.

I was okay with just doing my own thing for a while, push-ups and walks, waiting it out. Eventually, I slacked off. But as it became clear that gyms were not going to reopen anytime soon, I found that I did miss the pump you get from lifting weights, from supersets and reps to exhaustion, and even the ache from sore muscles the next day. I missed the pool, the exhilaration and meditation of swimming. And perhaps more than anything, the sense of community I'd always found in gyms, however small.

In New York State, gyms were allowed to reopen at the end of August 2020, more than five months after they had been shut down. Restrictions were put in place: A gym's capacity couldn't exceed one third; face masks and social distancing would be mandatory; temperature checks would be required upon entering. Equipment would have to be disinfected before and after each use, and gyms without sufficient air filtration systems would have to install them. Indoor pools were not yet allowed to reopen, however, nor were studios teaching group fitness classes, like spinning, yoga, and Pilates, as those settings were considered too dangerous in spreading Covid.

I waited until pools were allowed to reopen before I reactivated my membership at Chelsea Piers Fitness. But then I went on the very first day, September 30. The check-in desk was now just off the parking lot in the three-story warehouse-style building. Using an app the gym created, I scanned my membership bar code and submitted my "Daily Health Declaration," another of the new requirements. A staff person took my temperature, and I was allowed in.

I was nervous—not about catching Covid but about doing something wrong, inadvertently not following the new protocols. The place, usually so crowded, was vastly empty and quiet. The large restaurant that had filled the main space—once producing a near-constant roar of blenders, juicers, and human chatter—was shut down. Even the big-screen TVs were turned off. Making my way to the locker room, I had the same spooky feeling one has walking through an airport in the middle of the night. Large, illuminated signs had been posted. "NO SPOTTING," a few read, with a simple graphic of two hands crossed out with a big X.

No spotting: In two words, that phrase captured just how dramatically everything had changed. Spotting—physically interacting with other lifters, often total strangers, rooting them on, "C'mon, two more," as they went for a personal best—had once been a defining aspect of the unique microculture that is a gym. *Not* to spot—to turn someone down—or not to share equipment and weights would have been considered rude, unsportsmanlike, not long ago. Now they were considered high-risk behavior, a Covid-19 equivalent to the AIDS pandemic's unsafe sex.

I saw only two other men in the locker room, matched in number by masked janitors busily disinfecting surfaces—locker doors, bathroom counters, shower stalls. The sauna and spacious steam room were closed off indefinitely, perhaps forever, bringing to mind the crumbling, ancient baths, or *thermae*, that Mercuriale had found in Rome—ruins from another time, another culture. It was all so depressing. But I told myself not to dwell—to be grateful that I could even do this. I quickly changed into a swimsuit, grabbed a towel, and headed to the pool, right on time. You were told to be five minutes early. My swim reservation—thirty minutes, maximum—was for 2:10 P.M. I felt like I was going to a doctor's appointment.

The lifeguard confirmed my reservation and explained the rules: Wear your mask at all times, except for right before you get into the pool—he handed me a plastic sandwich bag to store it in at poolside. If you use a kickboard, pool buoy, or fins, he told me, hand them back to him afterward for disinfecting. Unlike in the past, each swimmer would have a lane to himself or herself—no lane sharing or circle swimming allowed—one of the few upsides to this pandemic. Although I was early, lane 1 was empty, and I could go ahead and swim.

Oliver's lane, I thought to myself: He always swam in lane 1. The lifeguard would even transfer swimmers from that lane to another just for him because that's where a ladder was located. (Oliver walked with a cane and couldn't crouch down and slip into the pool.) He always held tightly onto my arm as I guided him to the ladder, his huge flat feet flopping in swim fins, and helped him safely get in.

Now, I took off my mask, put on goggles, and plunged in.

The water was cold—cold! Not as cold as a mountain lake in October, but much colder than it had normally been. The pool must have been drained, cleaned, then refilled. *Oof!* I pushed off, hands outstretched in a V, legs doing a dolphin kick, until I surfaced about a third of the way down and launched into freestyle. My stroke immediately kicked in, as if not a day had passed since March. I had wondered if it would take time—time to find my rhythm, to synchronize bilateral breathing with crawling arms and legs—wondered if I would be rusty. But no, my body knew exactly what to do: thrust, pull, kick, rotate—swim. I touched the wall, flipped, pushed off. Lap after lap, I just swam, happy to forget about the pandemic and let my mind drift back.

On the Road to Olympia

It is a good thing to take journeys.

—ARETAEUS, CA. SECOND CENTURY A.D.

I had long dreamed of going to Olympia. I wanted to take a solo road trip like no other, searching for the sites of the ancient athletic games. This is something that Girolamo Mercuriale never had the opportunity to do. I almost felt that I owed it to him.

My first resource was not Fodor but Pindar, the ancient Greek lyric poet whose victory odes were written expressly for winners at athletic festivals. It was here I came to understand that Olympia was but one of four sites for the Panhellenic Games—contests open to athletes of the Greek, or Hellenic, Empire. In addition to the Olympics (then as now, held every four years), there were the Isthmian, Nemean, and Pythian Games in the intervals between. Going to all four sites was once a well-traveled circuit for athletes and spectators alike. Now, one cannot find Isthmia or Nemea described in many guidebooks.

I had sketched out my route over a beer in the bar at the American Academy in Rome. A young archaeologist there with strawberry-blonde hair told me how to get where I wanted to go—which was, in a sense, back in time 2,800 years. I had assumed that I could take trains from here to there, as I had in my travels throughout Italy. But no, the archaeologist explained, this would not work in Greece except in short stretches. Renting a car would make the most sense, and I could do a loop from one site to another, starting and ending in Athens. "Don't worry," she assured me, "once you get out of Athens the traffic is a cake walk."

Traffic wasn't what worried me. Traffic implies not driving, being stuck. It was the driving—fast, very fast, on the narrow, vertiginous roads I pictured—that had me concerned. But if a twenty-five-year-old can do it, someone more than twice her age can. So I booked a flight, a car, and hotels for four cities, and I got myself an International Driving Permit.

I SPENT TWO days in Athens before hitting the road. I'd been told several times that I would not like Athens, that it's "just a big city," like New York. But to say a place is like New York is the highest praise in my book, and I fell in love with Athens as immediately as I had with Manhattan. Athens in late June was very hot—perfect for air-conditioned museum going. I visited the new Acropolis Museum (ruins discovered during the museum's construction are visible beneath the entryway) and the National Archaeological Museum, a treasure trove of astonishing finds, including a few ancient strigils and the little clay pots used for storing gloios.

I got a good deal on a diesel-fuel, stick-shift car with Hertz. It didn't come equipped with GPS, but that was okay by me. Using GPS when you travel is like using performance-enhancing drugs in athletic competition, I believe. I'd rather go old school, I mean really old school, as in *The Odyssey*. Paper maps would get me where I wanted to go—I hoped.

I got out of Athens just fine, the car flying smoothly on the broad, multilane national highway. I caught myself smiling in the rearview mirror. Within ninety minutes, I was already spotting signs for Isthmia—so named for being on the Isthmus of Corinth, a narrow stretch of land connecting the mainland with the Peloponnese peninsula. To one side was the Gulf of Corinth, to the other, the Aegean Sea. I stopped at a gas station to ask for directions to the town.

"Isthmia?" said the clerk, a middle-aged woman in a bib apron. "Isthmia? This—Isthmia!"

"I'm in Isthmia?" Great, I replied, now where are the ancient ruins? She came out from behind the cash register and walked toward the window. Pointing west, she exclaimed, "Street? Yes!" Pause. "Bridge? Yes!" We locked eyes. Then she made that sound magicians make when they pull a rabbit out of a hat: poof! "Now, Isthmia!" And she was right, of course. Within minutes—poof!—I was pulling into a parking lot for the site of the ancient Isthmian ruins. There was no line. There was no crowd. There was no one else there, in fact, except the clerk, stray cats, and two large, unsmiling security guards. I stepped out into the blazing sun and surveyed the site—perhaps one hundred meters square.

I have to be honest: *forlorn* was the first word that came to mind. What Isthmia is today is mainly a dry field of rocks, dirt, and trees, only a fraction of which has been excavated by archaeologists. But forlorn is unfair, really, for this patch of earth remains rich with history. After all, Plato reportedly competed as a wrestler at the Isthmian Games as a young man in the early fifth century B.C. His sweat mixed with this dirt here on these very grounds. I took a handful and let it sprinkle from my palm.

I HAD TO get to Nemea by one P.M. that day. I had made an appointment well in advance with the distinguished archaeologist responsible for the Nemean excavations over the past thirty-five years, and he had just one hour to spare. I made it in time, barely, and found Dr. Stephen Miller at the entrance to one of the two main sites. We shook hands, and he strode ahead while launching into a history of Nemea as I scrambled for a pen. Stopping suddenly, he said, "We are in the locker room."

"Then this is the most beautiful locker room I've ever seen," I whispered. Nine fluted, sand-colored columns in varying heights stood with an air of majesty one senses in very rare creatures. The ground was even and smooth. On the perimeter: gardens, where wild rose bushes grew.

Dr. Miller explained that this was where athletes gathered before competition in the Nemean Games to undress and, as was the custom, to rub their bodies with olive oil and dust, which functioned as both a natural sunscreen and, not incidentally, an enhancer of muscular male beauty. They would then compete in the nude. "Now, back here," he continued, "is a 'secret entrance' we found from the locker room to the stadium." I followed him into a tunnel, about seven feet high and thirty yards long, with a remarkable vaulted ceiling—one of the earliest in recorded history. Some reconstruction had to be done to preserve the tunnel and render it safe for visitors, but evidence remained of its original use—and users. Miller pointed to some ancient Greek graffiti carved into the tunnel wall: "Akrotoos is beautiful," it read in translation.

"Wait, this is one man commenting on another?" I asked.

"Of course. Women were not allowed to compete in any of the athletic games," he explained, and only in certain specific instances were women even allowed to be spectators. Besides, sexual relationships between men were not uncommon at the time.

The stadium, six hundred feet long and wide enough to accommodate a dozen runners at a time, had been excavated to nearly pristine condition. The granite starting blocks remained firmly planted. Shallow ditches surrounding the entire area would have provided water from an aqueduct to moisten the dusty track between events—races of different lengths, as well as field events like the discus, javelin, and long jump. Wrestling, boxing, and the brutal ancient Greek equivalent to mixed martial arts, pankration, were also held here. Spectators watched from the gently sloping grass at the sides—about two thousand could be accommodated. A platform for judges, ancient-world arbiters for a photo-finish, was stationed at the end of the track.

From here, Dr. Miller said, we would go to the second site, a quarter mile down the road, where there was a temple dedicated to Zeus and other remains of the religious rituals held in conjunction with all the games. He suggested that I meet him there, and we both hopped into our cars. What happened next was inexplicable to me—in the moment, at least: a very loud bang, like a gunshot, and a feeling of being shoved. I saw in the rearview that the back window was completely shattered, but I had no idea why. Then I saw an olive tree trunk where a rear window should be. I had backed right into it at a fairly high speed, for I had the gear shift in reverse rather than in first, unintentionally. The back of the car was destroyed.

Dr. Miller pulled up beside me. "I've done that twice over the years," he called through his car window, "that damn tree—welcome to the club!" He chuckled, rolled up his window, and peeled off. There was nothing I could do about it now—Dr. Miller had only twenty minutes left, and the car did still work. I slowly rolled down the hill.

ONE SPLURGE I'D made on this trip was in buying all possible rental car insurance. After I placed a call from Nemea, Hertz had a replacement car waiting for me in Nafplio, a seaside town a couple of hours away, where I arranged to spend the night. I had to pay only a small deductible for the damage. This called for a celebratory swim. It was around six or six thirty, as I recall.

Thanos, the desk clerk at my small, family-run hotel, told me where I could go: to "a marble beach" on the other side of the jetty. I tried to get him to be specific about exactly where. "It's on the other side—" he pointed toward the door. "You'll find it."

Perhaps he didn't understand me. "How long does it take then?"

He shrugged his shoulders as if to indicate, it takes however long you wish.

I set out on a road that hugged the sea. The sun, near setting, still blazed at one hundred degrees. After about forty minutes, I did come to a marble beach. I had pictured it made from a million agates, in every color in a kaleidoscope—as if spilled from a goddess's pouch—but it was simply rocky. Though it was getting late, there were still people in the water. I watched for a while with an over-whelming feeling of calmness. The water looked black, like oil. The surf was fairly strong, waves crashing against the cement barriers. I shoved my clothes into a backpack and left it somewhere. I found a ladder on one of the barriers and lowered myself in, and I swam, I swam out far, and let the stresses of the day wash away.

The next morning, Thanos drew me a map of the route from Nafplio to Olympia: I would essentially traverse Peloponnese, east to west. He said it's very, very simple. He said the drive is very, very beautiful; it would take me maybe two hours. He also said he'd never done it before. By this point, I had derived a simple calculation for estimating how long it would take me to drive from one place to another, given my navigating abilities and propensity for getting lost: multiply by two and, for good measure, add an extra hour. So Thanos's "two hours to Olympia" would be, best-case scenario, five. Fine: I had a day to get to Olympia, I figured. Why not make a detour to see Mycenae then?

Mycenae was a fortified city on the Argolid plain, about an hour's drive north of Nafplio. Mycenaean civilization dates back nearly four thousand years, to the early Bronze Age. Among the earliest references to athletics originated here. Athletes held boxing and wrestling matches as entertainment (not competition per se) for the king. I had always imagined an enormous palace with an arena, but, once I had hiked up the hill where the palace ruins had been excavated, I realized that I had been mistaken. The king's palace was relatively small. Boxing opponents would have fought right in front of their king. He would have been able to smell the sweat on their bodies, hear bones crunching, and see, presumably to his satisfaction, men being pummeled to death a few feet away.

After retracing my route from Mycenae and getting back on the main route toward Olympia, I managed to get lost no less than three times, mainly because road signs were few and usually in Greek. Each time, a gas station attendant or store clerk helped me back on my way. Thanos was clearly a man of his word: The drive was very beautiful indeed, and getting more so the farther I ascended into the mountains.

At about the five-hour mark, I came upon a mountain village that was not marked on my maps. I parked and began walking around. One street wound through the small town. Above it and below, houses were built into the steep tree-covered mountainside, but I saw and heard no one. I felt that I had come upon a ghost-town Shangri-La.

I peeked into a restaurant (no one there) and a few shops (there neither) and kept walking until I came to a bar where a young couple, the proprietors, sat at a table on the sidewalk. He had the face and beard of a prehistoric warrior. She, luscious in a clingy summer dress, had copper-colored hair. They spoke very little English. I ordered two Coca-Colas and drank them in quick succession, I was so parched. I took out a map, and the young woman showed me where I was: in Arcadia, a word that's synonymous with utopia. Now I knew why.

On my way back to the car, I saw a man emerging from a restaurant, and I asked if it was open. "Sure," he answered in a mellow voice. He had a bushy beard and wore a Triumph motorcycle T-shirt. "I'll get you a menu." At that, he crossed the street and entered a different restaurant. I took a seat on the open-air patio, the lone diner there. He returned some minutes later. I ordered a beer. He turned and walked across the street. I loved this; no rush at all. Ten minutes later, maybe more, he was back with a frosty beer. I ordered a club sandwich.

"Tell me about this town," I asked. "What is the history?"

He looked uncomfortable. "My English is not good."

I assured him that was okay, and he told me a few small things. "It was built by builders," he said. "Workers who built houses for others in other towns." He said they came back here—kept the best spot for houses for themselves.

"Excellent. And you?"

"I came here about twenty years ago. Never left."

When the Triumph Man returned with my food a half hour later, I realized that he had made everything from scratch, including the fries. He then left me to eat—for so long that I assumed he had forgotten me. A thought passed through my mind that if I were to come back years from now and try to find this village, it would be gone, with no trace of the houses or the young couple or this restaurant. Before I left, I found the Triumph Man in the empty bar across the street. He smiled broadly, reached for a bottle, and poured a golden liquid into a small glass. He pushed it toward me.

"It's a Greek tradition," he said, answering the question on my face: a liqueur made from honey. He poured one for himself and we toasted. It was light and sweet, but not syrupy, stiff enough for two men to drink, as my dad would say.

He gave me a double espresso in a paper cup, and I paid my bill. I ducked my head back in just after exiting. "Olympia?" I said. "It's that way?" I pointed down the road.

"Yes, just down the road," he replied.

WHEN I PULLED into Olympia three hours later, eight since my drive had begun, I found the main street blocked with traffic at a standstill. I parked on a lower side street and walked toward the scene. A large crowd had converged around a shop with broken windows; there was glass on the sidewalk. It was a jewelry store, and a young man told me that armed bandits had robbed the store at gunpoint and grabbed the jewelry from the front window just minutes before. "Have they caught them?" I asked. The moment the words came out, I realized how naive that sounded.

"No one's going to get in the way of four men with guns," he scoffed. "People will do anything for money now in this country."

I left the scene, checked into my hotel, quickly got cleaned up, then hopped back into the car to visit the Olympic site before it closed at eight P.M.

As it turned out, this was a perfect time to go. Tour buses had left, and I found the site largely empty except for fifteen or twenty people. It was magically beautiful at dusk: hot—ninety degrees—but dry, the light of the low sun like liquid gold, and there were many trees to provide shade. The grounds, the size of about four football fields, were not cluttered with merchandise or souvenir stands, nor were guards everywhere admonishing you, as at so many of Italy's historic sites. One is left to oneself.

I visited the remains of the gymnasium, the stadium, the palestra, each exquisite in its simplicity and functionality. The serene, tranquil setting I wandered through had the feeling more of a religious retreat than a place where blood and sweat were spilled.

Many other buildings dotted the grounds, some of which were temples to gods and goddesses—the sanctuary to Zeus chief among them—some erected later (including a villa commissioned by a Roman emperor, who chose this piece of prime real estate). One has to use one's imagination to visually subtract those buildings that were not part of the original Olympics site, to envision what Olympia was like for athletes during the games. That was fine with me. Was it not imagination, a great collective imagination, which gave rise to the Olympic Games in the first place?

The traditional date given for the founding of the Olympics is 776 B.C., though historians now believe they may actually have started a little later. Regardless, the games held at Olympia were the earliest and longest surviving of Greek athletic festivals. One factor that made these games preeminent was a requirement for athletes at Olympia and Olympia alone: they had to pledge that they had trained for a minimum of ten successive months every year; and if so, they then trained together intensively for thirty days prior to the start of the games at a kind of camp nearby. This training was considered tougher than the Olympic Games themselves, effectively weeding out less-accomplished, less-dedicated athletes, and leaving the best of the best to compete. (This even comes up in the Bible: In one of St. Paul's letters to the Corinthians, he says of the need for self-discipline, "Everyone who competes in the [Olympic] games goes into strict training. They do it to get a crown that will not last, but we do it to get a crown that will last forever.") This organized year-round gym training—with the aim of keeping one's body in the best possible physical shape—was, in a sense, the progenitor of what today we would call working out.

I lingered at Olympia until the last possible moment, and thanked the two guards at the gate as I left. "It is so beautiful!" I couldn't help exclaiming.

One of the two, a woman, responded in broken English: "This is your job, you're here every day, you forget—"

"—how special it is?" I said.

"Yes," she smiled.

LEAVING OLYMPIA, I had a sense of freedom that I think of now as "being in fifth gear," the feeling, both literal and figurative, one has while cruising at top speed on a stretch of road, no cars in sight, the sea to the left, no worries. I stopped near Pyrgos, just before crossing the stunning new Rio–Antirrio Bridge, to get fuel and proper directions. I commented to the gas station attendant on how impressive the bridge looked from there.

The young man shook his head in disgust. "Yes, but—we are hungry here," he said. "That bridge: it's . . . false." By this, I gathered, he meant it's a sham the country could ill afford given the economy—a big spectacle, like the ancient statue of Zeus at Olympia, once one of the wonders of the world, or the overdesigned stadiums built for Olympic Games nowadays.

My itinerary for this trip had been dictated by geography—the easiest, fastest way to drive from one site to another—but as it turned out, there was an accidental chronological logic to it. Isthmia, my first stop, was the least excavated and developed, but the sites had gotten better as I went along, and I realized as I pulled into Delphi, home to the Pythian Games, that I may have saved the best for last.

The town is tucked into the southwestern spur of Mount Parnassus in the valley of Phocis, a spectacular setting. It was too late in the day to visit the site, but I caught a peek before sunset—truly breathtaking. I arrived at the site of the ancient ruins first thing the next morning. According to myth, the god Apollo started these games after he killed Python, the dragon residing here; hence, they were named the Pythian Games in recognition of this heroic act. In one important respect, the Pythian Games differed from those at Olympia, Nemea, and Isthmia: a competition for music and dance was held at the same time as the athletic games—an ancient Greek equivalent to *American Idol*-cum-*Dancing with the Stars*, so to speak.

I paused to get my bearings and apply sunblock before heading in—which is to say, up, for seeing this site involved a hike up the mountainside. I took my time walking toward the first major monument, the Temple of Apollo, as other visitors scurried past. I enjoyed soaking up the moment, having this gargantuan temple looming in my line of vision.

The temple itself was so large and solid it made the locker room at Nemea seem like a delicate miniature by comparison. I walked its perimeter and still found it hard to conceive how this had been built some three thousand years ago (slave labor is the answer, but something more, something mysterious in its architectural beauty, was also at play). Here at this temple is where the Oracle of Delphi resided. She—and it was always a she, a priestess—would inhale fumes rising from a crack in the earth (likely, gas emitting from natural mineral springs), which reportedly put her into a kind of trance, and she would prophesy events of the future.

It struck me that such a person could never predict all the unlikely places someone's wanderings could take them, on our planet and throughout history. No matter how psychically gifted, how empathetic, no seer could foretell how much a person's life might stretch them and test them, how much they might tear inside—or how much they might grow. I felt fortunate just to be there, to have made it to all four sites. I silently thanked Mercuriale for inspiring me. And as I began to make my ascent toward the theater and, farther up, to the stadium carved into the mountainside, a favorite passage from Pindar came to mind:

He who has achieved a new success
Basks in the light,
Soaring from hope to hope.
His deeds of prowess
Let him pace the air,
While he conceives
Plans sweeter to him than wealth.

ACKNOWLEDGMENTS

This book could not have been written without the generous support of the John Simon Guggenheim Foundation. I'm grateful to President Edward Hirsch and the Trustees of the foundation for their belief in this project, and to the Leon Levy Foundation for providing supplemental funding to my fellowship. I'd also like to express gratitude to the American Academy in Rome and to Blue Mountain Center, both of which provided residencies for research and writing.

Very special thanks to Arlene Shaner, who introduced me to Girolamo Mercuriale and provided crucial research assistance, advice, and encouragement throughout the writing of this book. I'm also grateful to Jean-Michel Agasse, Giancarlo Cerasoli, and Vivian Nutton for so generously sharing their research and insights with me. Many thanks as well to Steven Barclay, Peter Catapano, Carlyle David, Emily Forland, Lisa Garrigues, Ben Hyman, Myunghee Kwon, Harriet LeFavour, David Mann, Dawn McInnis, Nancy Miller, Laura Phillips, Alessandro Pisoni, Alexandra Pringle, and Patti Ratchford.

BIBLIOGRAPHY

BOOKS AND ARTICLES

Agasse, Jean-Michel. "Girolamo Mercuriale: Humanism and Physical Culture in the Renaissance." Translated from French by Christine Nutton. In Mercuriale, *Girolamo Mercuriale: De arte gymnastica*, 861–1118. English-language translation of Mercuriale's text included. Translated from Latin by Vivian Nutton. Florence, Italy: Leo S. Olschki, 2008.

Ananthaswamy, Anil. "The Exercise Paradox." *New Scientist*, June 1, 2013, 28–29.

Angelopoulou, N., et al. "Hippocrates on Health and Exercise." *Nikephoros* 13 (2000): 141–52.

Arcangeli, Alessandro, and Vivian Nutton, eds. *Girolamo Mercuriale: Medicina e cultura nell'Europa del cinquecento*. Florence, Italy: Leo S. Olschki, 2008.

Aristotle. *Problems: Books 1–19*. Translated by Robert Mayhew. Cambridge, MA: Harvard University Press, 2011.

Aristotle. *Problems: Books 20–38*. Translated by Robert Mayhew. Cambridge, MA: Harvard University Press, 2011.

Aschwanden, Christie. "Faster Body, Faster Mind." *New Scientist*, November 9, 2013, 44–47.

Barry, John M. *The Great Influenza*. New York: Penguin Books, 2004.

Beecher, Catharine. *A Treatise on Domestic Economy*. New York: Harper & Bros., 1848.

Berryman, Jack W., and Robert J. Park, eds. *Sport and Exercise Science: Essays in the History of Sports Medicine*. Urbana: University of Illinois Press, 1992.

Biagioli, Brian D. *Advanced Concepts of Personal Training*. Coral Gables, FL: National Council on Strength & Fitness, 2007.

Black, Jonathan. *Making the American Body*. Lincoln: University of Nebraska Press, 2013.

Blasé, Irene. Unpublished translation of Girolamo Mercuriale's *De decoratione liber* (Venice, Italy: Giunta, 1585). Collection of Clendening History of Medicine Library, University of Kansas Medical Center, Kansas City.

Blasé, Irene. Unpublished translation of Girolamo Mercuriale's *De excrementis* (Venice, Italy: Giunta, 1572). Collection of Clendening History of Medicine Library, University of Kansas Medical Center, Kansas City.

Borelli, Giovanni Alfonso. *De motu animalium*. Rome: Angeli Bernabó, 1680–81.

Bowie, Ewen, and Jas Elsner, eds. *Philostratus*. Cambridge, UK: Cambridge University Press, 2009.

Brailsford, Dennis. *British Sport: A Social History*. Rev. ed. Cambridge, UK: Lutterworth Press, 1997.

Bramble, Dennis M., and Daniel E. Lieberman. "Endurance Running and the Evolution of *Homo*." *Nature*, November 18, 2014, 345–52.

Brod, Max. *Franz Kafka: A Biography*. Translated by G. Humphrey Roberts and Richard Winston. New York: Schocken Books, 1960.

Butler, George. *Arnold Schwarzenegger: A Portrait*. New York: Simon & Schuster, 1990.

Castiglione, Baldesar. *The Book of the Courtier*. Translated by George Bull. New York: Penguin Books, 1967.

Celenza, Christopher S. *The Lost Italian Renaissance*. Baltimore: Johns Hopkins University Press, 2004.

Christensen, Paul, and Donald G. Kyle, eds. *A Companion to Sport and Spectacle in Greek and Roman Antiquity*. Hoboken, NJ: Wiley Blackwell, 2014.

Coffin, David R. *Pirro Ligorio: The Renaissance Artist, Architect, and Antiquarian*. University Park: Pennsylvania State University Press, 2004.

Cohen, Elizabeth S., and Timothy Cohen. *Daily Life in Renaissance Italy*. Westport, CT: Greenwood Press, 2001.

Conrad, Lawrence I., Michael Neve, Vivian Nutton, Roy Porter, and Andrew Wear. *The Western Medical Tradition: 800 B.C.–1800 A.D.* Cambridge, UK: Cambridge University Press, 1995.

Corcoran, Clinton. "Wrestling and the Fair Fight in Plato." *Nikephoros* 16 (2003): 61–85.

Corvisier, Jean-Nicolas. "Hygieia: Plutarch's Views on Good Health." *Nikephoros* 16 (2003): 115–46.

Crowther, Nigel B. "The Olympic Training Period." *Nikephoros* 4 (1991): 161–66.

Crowther, Nigel B. "The Palestra, Gymnasium, and Physical Exercise in Cicero." *Nikephoros* 15 (2002): 159–74.

Decker, Wolfgang. *Sports and Games of Ancient Egypt.* Translated by Allen Guttmann. New Haven, CT: Yale University Press, 1992.

Delavier, Frederic. *Strength Training Anatomy.* Champaign, IL: Human Kinetics, 2010.

Dickie, Matthew W. "Calisthenics in the Greek and Roman Gymnasium." *Nikephoros* 6 (1993): 105–51.

Dimon, Theodore. *The Body in Motion: Its Evolution and Design.* Berkeley, CA: North Atlantic Books, 2011.

Duby, Georges, ed. *Revelations of the Medieval World.* Vol. 2 of *A History of Private Life.* Translated by Arthur Goldhammer. Cambridge, MA: Belknap Press of Harvard University Press, 1988.

Dutton, Kenneth R. *The Perfectible Body: The Western Ideal of Male Physical Development.* New York: Continuum, 1995.

Evans, Nick. *Bodybuilding Anatomy.* Champaign, IL: Human Kinetics, 2007.

Ferretti, Anna Colombi. *Il complesso monumentale di San Mercuriale a Forlì Restauri.* Forlì-Cesena, Italy: STC Group, 2000.

Folk, G. Edgar, and Holmes A. Semken Jr. "The Evolution of Sweat Glands." *International Journal of Biometeorology* 35 (1991): 180–86.

Fonda, Jane. *Jane Fonda's Workout.* VHS. Produced by Sid Galanty. Released by Karl Home Video and RCA Video Productions, 1982.

Fonda, Jane. *Jane Fonda's Workout Book.* New York: Simon & Schuster, 1981.

Fonda, Jane. *My Life So Far.* New York: Random House, 2005.

Fuller, Francis. *Medicina Gymnastica, or, A Treatise Concerning the Power of Exercise.* London: printed by John Matthews at the *Angel and Crown* in St. Paul's Church, 1705.

Gage, Frances. "Exercise for Mind and Body: Giulio Mancini, Collecting, and the Beholding of Landscape Painting in the Seventeenth Century." *Renaissance Quarterly* 61 (2008): 1167–207.

Gaines, Charles, and George Butler. *Pumping Iron: The Art and Sport of Bodybuilding.* New York: Simon & Schuster, 1974.

Galen. *Galen's Hygiene (De Sanitate Tuenda).* Translated by Robert Montraville Green, MD. Springfield, IL: Charles C. Thomas, 1951.

Galen. *Selected Works.* Translated by P. N. Singer. New York: Oxford University Press, 1997.

Gallini, Giovanni Andrea. *A Treatise on the Art of Dancing.* London: printed for the author, 1762.

Gamrath, Helge. *Farnese: Pomp, Power, and Politics in Renaissance Italy.* Rome: L'Erma di Bretschneider, 2007.

Gardiner, E. Norman. *Athletics of the Ancient World.* London: Oxford University Press, 1971.

Gaston, Robert W. *Pirro Ligorio: Artist and Antiquarian.* Milan: Silvana Editoriale, 1988.

Gay, Peter. *Freud: A Life for Our Times.* New York: W. W. Norton, 1988.

Georgii, Carl August. *Kinetic Jottings: Miscellaneous Extracts from Medical Literature, Ancient and Modern.* London: Henry Renshaw, 1880.

Gerber, Ellen W. *Innovators and Institutions in Physical Education.* Philadelphia: Lea & Febiger, 1971.

Goethe, Johann Wolfgang. *Maxims and Reflections.* Translated by Elisabeth Stopp. New York: Penguin Books, 1998.

Golden, Mark. *Sport and Society in Ancient Greece.* Cambridge, UK: Cambridge University Press, 1998.

Goldstein, Richard. "Jack LaLanne, Founder of Modern Fitness Movement, Dies at Ninety-Six." *New York Times,* January 24, 2011.

Grafton, Anthony, ed. *Rome Reborn: The Vatican Library and Renaissance Culture.* Washington, DC: Library of Congress, 1993.

Grafton, Anthony, Glenn W. Most, and Salvatore Settis, eds. *The Classical Tradition.* Cambridge, MA: Belknap Press of Harvard University Press, 2010.

Green, Harvey. *Fit for America: Health, Fitness, Sport, and American Society.* New York: Pantheon Books, 1986.

Gutsmuths, Johann Christoph Friedrich. *Gymnastik für die Jugend.* Schnepfenthal, Germany: Buchhandlung der Erziehungsanstalt, 1793.

Guttmann, Allen. *The Erotic in Sports.* New York: Columbia University Press, 1996.

Hagelin, Ova. *Kinetic Jottings: Rare and Curious Books in the Library of the Old Royal Central Institute of Gymnastics.* Stockholm, Sweden: Hagelin Rare Books AB, 1995.

Hamill, Joseph, and Kathleen M. Knutzen. *Biomechanical Basis of Human Movement.* 3rd ed. Baltimore: Lippincott Williams & Wilkins, 2009.

Harris, H. A. *Sport in Greece and Rome.* London: Thames and Hudson, 1979.

Harvey, William. *De motu locali animalium, 1627.* Translated by Gweneth Whitteridge. Cambridge, UK: Cambridge University Press, 1959.

Hecht, Jennifer Michael. *The Happiness Myth: Why What We Think Is Right Is Wrong.* New York: Harper Collins, 2007.

Herlihy, David V. *Bicycle.* New Haven, CT: Yale University Press, 2004.

Hesiod. *Works and Days.* Translated by Glenn W. Most. Cambridge, MA: Harvard University Press, 2018.

Hippocrates. *The Medical Works of Hippocrates*. Translated by John Chadwick and W. N. Mann. Oxford, UK: Blackwell Scientific Publications, 1950.

Hippocrates. *Regimen in Health. Regimen 1–3*. Translated by W. H. S. Jones. Loeb Classical Library 150. Cambridge, MA: Harvard University Press, 1931.

Homer. *The Iliad*. Translated by Stephen Mitchell. New York: Free Press, 2011.

Homer. *The Odyssey*. Translated by Robert Fagles. New York: Penguin Classics, Deluxe Edition, 1996.

Horstmanshoff, Manfred, Helen King, and Claus Zittel, eds. *Blood, Sweat, and Tears: The Changing Concepts of Physiology from Antiquity into Early Modern Europe*. Leiden, Netherlands: Brill, 2012.

Howell, Maxwell L. *People's Republic of China Four-Minute Exercise Plan*. New York: Grosset & Dunlap, 1973.

Huizinga, Johan. *Homo Ludens: A Study of the Play Element in Culture*. Boston: Beacon, 1972.

Jahn, Friedrich Ludwig. *Treatise on Gymnastics*. Translated by Charles Butler. Northampton, MA: Simeon Butler, 1828.

Joyce, James. *Ulysses: The Complete and Unabridged Text*. New York: Vintage International, 1990.

Kafka, Franz. *The Diaries of Franz Kafka, Volume Two: 1914–1923*. Translated by Martin Greenberg and Hannah Arendt. London: Secker & Warburg, 1949.

Kraus, Hans, and Ruth P. Hirschland. "Muscular Fitness and Health." *Journal of the American Association for Health, Physical Education, and Recreation* 24, no. 10 (1953): 17–19.

Kuno, Yas. *Human Perspiration*. Springfield, IL: Charles C. Thomas, 1956.

Kyle, Donald G. *Sport and Spectacle in Ancient Greece*. Malden, MA: Blackwell, 2007.

Laden, Karl, ed. *Antiperspirants and Deodorants*. New York: Marcel Dekker, 1999.

Laughlin, Terry. *Total Immersion: The Revolutionary Way to Swim Better, Faster, and Easier.* New York: Fireside, 2004.

Lee, Hugh M. "The *caestus* in the Sixteenth Century: Brant, Raphael, Mercuriale, and Ligorio." *Nikephoros* 18 (2005): 207–17.

Lee, Hugh M. "Girolamo Mercuriale: De Arte Gymnastica." *Nikephoros* 22 (2009): 263–71.

Lee, Hugh M. "Mercuriale, Ligorio, and the Revival of Greek Sports in the Renaissance." In *Cultural Relations Old and New: The Transitory Olympic Ethos.* London, ON: International Centre for Olympic Studies, 2004.

Leonard, Fred Eugene. *Pioneers of Modern Physical Training.* New York: Association Press, 1922.

Lewis, Diocletian. *The New Gymnastics for Men, Women, and Children.* Boston: Ticknor & Fields, 1862–68.

Ling, Pehr Henrik. *Gymnastikens Allmänna Grunder.* Upsala, Sweden: Leffler & Sebell, 1840.

Lo, Vivienne. *Perfect Bodies: Sports, Medicine, and Immortality.* London: British Museum, 2012.

Locke, John. *Some Thoughts Concerning Education.* London: 1693.

Löfving, Concordia. *On Physical Education, and Its Place in a Rational System of Education.* London: W. Swan Sonnenschein, 1882.

Mann, Thomas. *Essays.* Translated by H. T. Lowe-Porter. New York: Vintage Books, 1957.

Mantas, Konstantinos. "Women and Athletics in the Roman East." *Nikephoros* 8 (1995): 125–44.

Massengale, John D., and Richard A. Swanson, eds. *The History of Exercise and Sport Science.* Champaign, IL: Human Kinetics, 1997.

Mattern, Susan P. *The Prince of Medicine: Galen in the Roman Empire.* New York: Oxford University Press, 2013.

McClelland, John. *Body and Mind: Sport in Europe from the Roman Empire to the Renaissance.* New York: Routledge, 2007.

McDougall, Christopher. *Born to Run: A Hidden Tribe, Superathletes, and the Greatest Race the World Has Never Seen.* New York: Vintage Books, 2011.

McGinn, Colin. *Sport.* Stocksfield, UK: Acumen, 2008.

McKenzie, Shelly. *Getting Physical: The Rise of Fitness Culture in America.* Lawrence: University Press of Kansas, 2013.

Mechikoff, Robert A., and Steven G. Estes. *A History and Philosophy of Sport and Physical Education from Ancient Civilization to the Modern World.* New York: McGraw-Hill, 1993.

Mendez, Christobal. *Book of Bodily Exercise.* Translated by Francisco Guerra. New Haven, CT: Elizabeth Licht, 1960.

Mercuriale, Girolamo. *De arte gymnastica.* Venice, Italy: Giunta, 1569 (first edition) and 1573 (second edition).

Mercuriale, Girolamo. *De decoratione liber.* Venice, Italy: Giunta, 1585.

Mercuriale, Girolamo. *De morbis cutaneis, et omnibus corporis humani excrementis tractatus locupletissimi . . .* Venice, Italy: Giunta, 1572.

Mercuriale, Girolamo. *De pestilentia.* Venice, Italy: Giunta, 1577.

Mercuriale, Girolamo. *Girolamo Mercuriale: De arte gymnastica.* Translated from Latin by Vivian Nutton. Florence, Italy: Leo S. Olschki, 2008.

Mercuriale, Girolamo. *Nomothelasmus.* Padua, Italy: Giacomo Fabriano, 1552.

Miller, Stephen G. *The Ancient Stadium of Nemea.* Walnut Creek, CA: Thomas J. Long Foundation, n.d.

Miller, Stephen G. *Arete: Greek Sports from Ancient Sources.* Berkeley: University of California Press, 2004.

Mondschein, Ken. *The Knightly Art of Battle.* Los Angeles: J. Paul Getty Museum, 2011.

Morris, Jeremy, et al. "Coronary Heart Disease and Physical Activity of Work." *The Lancet* 262 (November 21, 1953): 1053–57.

Mulcaster, Richard. *Positions*. London: printed by Thomas Vautrollier for Thomas Chare, 1581.

Neils, Jenifer. *Goddess and Polis: The Panathenaic Festival in Ancient Athens*. Hanover, NH: Hood Museum of Art, Dartmouth College, 1992.

Nutton, Christine. "Mercurialis's Life and Work." In *Hieronymus Mercurialis, De arte gymnastica*. Stuttgart, Germany: Edition Medicina Rara, 1978.

Nutton, Vivian, ed. *Medicine at the Courts of Europe, 1500–1837*. Abingdon, UK: Routledge, 1990.

Nutton, Vivian. "The Pleasures of Erudition: Mercuriale's *Variae Lectiones*." In *Girolamo Mercuriale: Medicina e cultura nell'Europa del cinquecento*, edited by Alessandro Arcangeli and Vivian Nutton, 77–95. Florence, Italy: Leo S. Olschki, 2008.

Oates, Joyce Carol. *On Boxing*. Updated and expanded ed. New York: Harper Perennial, 2006.

Palmer, Richard. "Girolamo Mercuriale and the Plague of Venice." In *Girolamo Mercuriale: Medicina e cultura nell'Europa del cinquecento*, edited by Alessandro Arcangeli and Vivian Nutton, 51–65. Florence, Italy: Leo S. Olschki, 2008.

Panvinio, Onofrio. *De ludis circensibus*. 2nd ed. Padua, Italy: Pauli Frambotti, 1642.

Park, Katharine. *Doctors and Medicine in Early Renaissance Florence*. Princeton, NJ: Princeton University Press, 1985.

Partner, Peter. *Renaissance Rome, 1500–1559: A Portrait of a Society*. Berkeley: University of California Press, 1976.

Pascha, Johann Georg. *Gründliche Beschreibung des Voltiger*. Halle, Germany: Melchior Oelschlegel, 1666.

Philostratus. *Heroicus, Gymnasticus, Discourses 1 and 2*. Translated by Jeffrey Rusten and Jason König. Cambridge, MA: Harvard University Press, 2014.

Pindar. *Pindar's Victory Songs*. Translated by Frank J. Nisetich. Baltimore: Johns Hopkins University Press, 1980.

Piranonmonte, Marina. *The Baths of Caracalla*. Milan: Mondadori Electa, 2008.

Plato. *Plato: The Man and His Work*. Translated by A. E. Taylor. Mineola, NY: Dover Publications, 2001 (unaltered republication of the fourth edition originally published in 1926 by Methuen, London).

Plato. *The Republic of Plato*. Translated by Francis MacDonald Cornford. London: Oxford University Press, 1951.

Pleket, H. W. "The Infrastructure of Sport in the Cities of the Greek World." *Scienze dell'antichita: Storia, archeologia, antropologia* 10: 627–44.

Pleket, H. W. "Roman Emperors and Greek Athletes." *Nikephoros* 23 (2010): 175–203.

Porter, Roy. *Flesh in the Age of Reason: The Modern Foundations of Body and Soul*. New York: W. W. Norton, 2004.

Potter, David. *The Victor's Crown: A History of Ancient Sport from Homer to Byzantium*. New York: Oxford University Press, 2012.

Powers, Scott K., and Edward T. Howley. *Exercise Physiology: Theory and Application to Fitness and Performance*. 8th ed. New York: McGraw Hill, 2012.

President's Council on Physical Fitness. *Adult Physical Fitness: A Program for Men and Women*. Washington, DC: US Government Printing Office, ca. 1962.

Quinn, Susan. *Marie Curie: A Life*. New York: Simon & Schuster, 1995.

Remijsen, Sofie. *The End of Greek Athletics in Late Antiquity*. Cambridge, UK: Cambridge University Press, 2015.

Renbourn, E. T. "The History of Sweat and the Sweat Rash from Earliest Times to the End of the Eighteenth Century." *Journal of the History of Medicine* 9 (April 1959): 202–27.

Rifkin, Benjamin A., and Michael J. Ackerman. *Human Anatomy: From the Renaissance to the Digital Age*. New York: Harry N. Abrams, 2006.

Robertson, Claire. *Il Gran Cardinale: Alessandro Farnese, Patron of the Arts.* New Haven, CT: Yale University Press, 1992.

Rousseau, Jean-Jacques. *Emile, or On Education.* Translated by Allan Bloom. New York: Basic Books, 1979.

Sandow, Eugen. *Strength and How to Obtain It.* London: Gale & Polden, 1897.

Santorio, Santorio. *Medicina Statica: Being the Aphorisms of Sanctorius.* Translated by John Quincy. London: W. J. Newton et al., 1723–24.

Scanlon, Thomas F. *Eros and Greek Athletics.* New York: Oxford University Press, 2002.

Singleton, Mark. *Yoga Body: The Origins of Modern Posture Practice.* New York: Oxford University Press, 2010.

Siraisi, Nancy G. *Communities of Learned Experience.* Baltimore: Johns Hopkins University Press, 2013.

Siraisi, Nancy G. "History, Antiquarianism, and Medicine: The Case of Girolamo Mercuriale." *Journal of the History of Ideas* 64 (April 2003): 231–51.

Siraisi, Nancy G. *Medieval and Early Renaissance Medicine: An Introduction to Knowledge and Practice.* Chicago: University of Chicago Press, 1990.

Siraisi, Nancy G. "Mercuriale's Letters to Zwinger and Humanist Medicine." In *Girolamo Mercuriale: Medicina e cultura nell'Europa del cinquecento*, edited by Alessandro Arcangeli and Vivian Nutton, 77–95. Florence, Italy: Leo S. Olschki, 2008.

Solari, Giovanna R. *The House of Farnese: A Portrait of a Great Family of the Renaissance.* Translated by Simona Morini and Frederic Tuten. Garden City, NY: Doubleday, 1968.

Spears, Betty. "A Perspective of the History of Women's Sport in Ancient Greece." *Journal of Sport History* 11, no. 2 (Summer 1984): 32-47.

Sutton, Richard L. *Sixteenth Century Physician and His Methods: Mercurialis on Diseases of the Skin.* Kansas City, MO: Lowell Press, 1986.

Sweet, Waldo. *Sport and Recreation in Ancient Greece.* New York: Oxford University Press, 1987.

Syman, Stefanie. *The Subtle Body: The Story of Yoga in America.* New York: Farrar, Straus and Giroux, 2010.

Thibault d'Anvers, Gérard. *Academie de l'Espée.* Leiden, Netherlands: Elzevir, 1628–30.

Tipton, Charles M., ed. *Exercise Physiology: People and Ideas.* New York: Oxford University Press, 2003.

Todd, Jan. "From Milo to Milo: A History of Barbells, Dumbbells, and Indian Clubs." *Iron Game History* 3, no. 6 (1995): 4–16.

Todd, Jan. *Physical Culture and the Body Beautiful: Purposive Exercise in the Lives of American Women, 1800–1875.* Macon, GA: Mercer University Press, 1998.

Tuccaro, Archangelo. *Trois dialogues de l'exercise de sauter et voltiger en l'air.* Paris: Claude de Monstr'oeil: 1599.

Tyrrell, William Blake. *The Smell of Sweat: Greek Athletics, Olympics, and Culture.* Wauconda, IL: Bolchazy-Carducci, 2004.

Vagenheim, Ginette. "Pirro Ligorio." In *Encyclopedia of the Renaissance,* edited by Paul F. Grendler. Vol. 3. New York: Charles Scribner's Sons, 1999.

Vegetius, Publius Flavius Renatus. *De rei militari libri.* Leiden, Netherlands: Plantin Press, 1607.

Vella, Mark. *Anatomy for Strength and Fitness Training.* New York: McGraw Hill, 2006.

Vertinsky, Patricia A. *The Eternally Wounded Woman: Women, Doctors, and Exercise in the Late Nineteenth Century.* Urbana: University of Illinois Press, 1994.

Veyne, Paul, ed. *From Pagan Rome to Byzantium.* Vol. 1 of *A History of Private Life.* Translated by Arthur Goldhammer. Cambridge, MA: Belknap Press of Harvard University Press, 1987.

Vigarello, Georges. *The Metamorphosis of Fat: A History of Obesity*. Translated by C. Jon Delogu. New York: Columbia University Press, 2013.

Waddy, Patricia. *Seventeenth-Century Roman Palaces: Use and the Art of the Plan*. Cambridge, MA: MIT Press, 1990.

Waller, David. *The Perfect Man: The Muscular Life and Times of Eugen Sandow, Victorian Strongman*. Brighton, UK: Victorian Secrets, 2011.

West, Michael. "Everard Digby, and the Renaissance Art of Swimming." *Renaissance Quarterly* 26, no. 1 (1973): 11–22.

Zander, Gustaf. *Dr. G. Zander's Medico-Mechanische Gymnastik*. Stockholm, Sweden: P. A. Norstedt & Söner, 1892.

Zeigler, Earle F. *History of Physical Education and Sport*. Champaign, IL: Stipes, 1988.

Zeigler, Earle F. *Sport and Physical Education in the Middle Ages*. Bloomington, IN: Trafford, 2006.

WEBSITES

"Alessandro Farnese." Wikipedia. en.wikipedia.org/wiki/Alessandro _Farnese. Accessed July 5, 2013.

"Alfonso II d'Este, Duke of Ferrara." Wikipedia. en.wikipedia.org/wiki /Alfonso_II_d%27Este,_Duke_of_Ferrara. Accessed April 3, 2014.

Brouwers, Josho. "Roman Girls in 'Bikinis'—A Mosaic from the Villa Romana del Casale." Ancient World Magazine. https://www.ancient worldmagazine.com/articles/roman-girls-bikinis-mosaic-villa-romana -del-casale-sicily/. Accessed April 2021.

"Council of Trent, Session XXV, On Reformation, Eighth Decree, Chapter XIX [On dueling]." The Council of Trent. http://www.thecounciloftrent .com/ch25.htm. Accessed April 2021.

"Gerard Thibault d'Anvers." Wikipedia. en.wikipedia.org/wiki/G%C3 %A9rard_Thibault_d%27Anvers. Accessed May 28, 2014.

"Girolamo Mercuriale." Wikipedia. en.wikipedia.org/wiki/Girolamo _Mercuriale. Accessed July 5, 2013.

"History of Fencing." Wikipedia. en.wikipedia.org/wiki/History_of _fencing. Accessed May 28, 2014.

"Onofrio Panvinio." Wikipedia. en.wikipedia.org/wiki/Onofrio_Panvinio. Accessed July 5, 2013.

"Pirro Ligorio." Wikipedia. en.wikipedia.org/wiki/Pirro_Ligorio. Accessed April 3, 2014.

"Pope Pius IV." Wikipedia. en.wikipedia.org/wiki/Pope_Pius_VI. Accessed July 14, 2013.

"President's Council on Sports, Fitness & Nutrition—History." US Department of Health and Human Services. www.hhs.gov/fitness/about -pcsfn/our-history/index.html. Accessed December 2020.

Sturgeon, Julie, and Janice Meer. "The First Fifty Years: 1956–2006." US Department of Health and Human Services. www.hhs.gov/sites/default /files/fitness/pdfs/50-year-anniversary-booklet.pdf. Accessed December 2020.

Thayer, Bill. "Vitruvius: On Architecture." penelope.uchicago.edu/Thayer/e /roman/texts/vitruvius/home.html. Accessed January 2021.

Wilson-Barlow, Lindsay. "The Physiological Effects of Laughter." www .findapsychologist.org/the-physiological-effects-of-laughter-by-lindsay -wilson-barlow/. Accessed December 2020.

INDEX

A NOTE ON THE AUTHOR

Bill Hayes is the author of *How We Live Now*, *Insomniac City*, and *The Anatomist*, among other books. Hayes is a recipient of a Guggenheim Fellowship in nonfiction and is a frequent contributor to the *New York Times*. A collection of his street photography, *How New York Breaks Your Heart*, was published recently by Bloomsbury. Hayes has completed the screenplay for a film adaptation of *Insomniac City*, currently in the works from Brouhaha Entertainment, and he is also a coeditor of Oliver Sacks's posthumous books. He lives in New York. Visit his website at billhayes.com.